Fit for Success

Joan Geraghty

First published in 2009 by
CURRACH PRESS
55A Spruce Avenue, Stillorgan Industrial Park, Blackrock, Co. Dublin
www.currach.ie

1 3 5 4 2

Cover by bluett
Origination by Currach Press
Printed in Ireland by ColourBooks, Baldoyle Industrial Estate, Dublin 13
ISBN:978-1-85607-981-5

Acknowledgements

I wish to thank Jo O'Donoghue of Currach Press for backing me with this, my second book; for letting me just get on with it and trusting me to produce the goods.

Thanks also to all the interviewees in the book, who generously gave of their time and energy to share their wisdom and experience of fitness and success.

A special word of gratitude to my parents, Richard and Beda Tobin, for forgetting to teach me how to grow old and for showing the world that age really is just a number.

To the good Lord above, I wish to express my gratitude for sparing the life of my husband Padraic, so that he can remain a dad to our small children. Padraic recently had triple-by-pass heart surgery.

To all the Geraghtys for their fabulous support throughout our ordeal and to all my own gang, the Tobins, the Pierses in Tipperary, all our colleagues in the *Mayo News* and the people of Westport and Castlebar, for their care and concern.

Finally, warm tributes to the staff of Mayo General Hospital, the A&E and Intensive Care Units and the Coronary Care surgery and nursing staff at University College Hospital Galway and to Croi West of Ireland Cardiology Foundation for the wonderful work they do for heart patients and their families.

Thank you all so much.

Joan Geraghty, Westport, March 2009

*This book is dedicated to all those who want
to improve the quality of their lives
and who are prepared to make the effort to do so.*

Contents

INTRODUCTION

It may seem like a coincidence that some of the most successful people in business also happen to be in top shape but these two factors – fitness and success – may well be inextricably linked. Of course it's not a given that you must be fit in order to be successful at your work but certainly – as some of the inspiring interviewees in this book attest – fitness helps.

I immersed myself in the fitness world three years ago and can now vouch for the fact that physical fitness is a truly powerful tool for building success. Starting off as a non-runner, I graduated to becoming a marathon runner, with the result that challenging exercise is now standard in my life.

In the process, I have become more ambitious, more productive and more driven – ready to turn my hand to whatever life throws at me. During good times and bad, keeping fit makes me positive and upbeat. It's like having a constant supply of feel-good helpers to call on, with every workout providing a new 'can do' hit.

People who love working out, building up their muscle mass, breaking into sweats – all in the name of fitness – subscribe to the view that it is exercise that keeps them on top of their game. This is because exercise makes you feel good about yourself and how you are using your body, which in turn fires up your self-confidence, helping you to do the work you want to do.

Nor do you have to engage in hard-core exercise in order to enjoy the energy boost and mental clarity that come from working out. Adherents of Eastern fitness and martial arts disciplines, such as yoga, pilates, tai chi and tak wan doo, as well as those who practise meditation or regularly commune with nature, are often totally focused individuals, motivated to reach their highest potential.

In essence, people who succeed in life usually show discipline with regard to how they work and how they choose to live. Applying that same discipline to their fitness regime, by dedicating a certain, minimum amount of time daily or weekly to practising an art or exercise that gives them ongoing pleasure evidently heightens their potential for success.

My first book, *Anyone Can Run*, dealt a lot with the fantastic benefits running confers on a body. I particularly recall my idol, Professor Risteárd Mulcahy, (whose book, *Improving with Age*, was probably responsible for getting me interested in fitness in the first place), waxing lyrical about the spiritual and physical highs that come from consistent running training.

Running was a great joy in Professor Mulcahy's life, even though he was almost sixty before he really became involved in it. When physical decline forced him to give up running at the age of seventy-four, he talked sadly about how he still yearned to follow younger runners on their workouts and, like them, achieve the famous 'runner's high'.

It is now clear to me that running is just one pathway to achieving the after-glow that comes from hard workouts and consistent training. The people I spoke to in this book show that other sports and disciplines, when practised with dedication, can confer similar physical and mental benefits

– be they individual pursuits such as boxing or mountain climbing, or team sports such as basketball or hockey.

In *Anyone Can Run* I documented the phenomenal impact taking up running at the age of forty had on my life. After the book was published, I managed to continue my running training, building up to running my first marathon in Connemara in April 2008. That experience was life-changing, proving to me that training in accordance with a programme can really deliver results. It also made me think that anyone who can run can also run a marathon. But that's a book for another day.

(A full report on my Connemara marathon run, which I completed in four hours and fourteen minutes, can be found on my blog – anyonecanrun.blogspot.com – as well as on my e-fitness magazine, fitnessjunkie.ie.)

The Dublin Adidas Marathon 2008 was my second marathon (four hours sixteen minutes) and since then my fitness and running training have taken on a completely different character. I would no longer describe myself as a plodder. Running is no longer just about getting out there and doing it. It's about getting out there and pushing myself hard and sometimes very hard. I find that this more challenging approach gives me greater natural highs than ever. Working out is one thing but really pushing the body, taking it through the sheer hell of hard physical demands, is amazing. The body loves it, I swear!

At the same time, I am not, nor am I trying to be, a competitive or winning athlete. This doesn't mean that I can't run faster than I do at the moment, nor that I can't go on achieving new personal bests. What has become clear to me now – with a certain level of fitness already in the bag

– is that working out as hard as I can, as opposed to just regularly working out, makes me feel totally on top of my game. Challenging my body to achieve more and continually upping the ante on my personal goals is making me happier in my own skin, my own body, than I have ever been before.

It's as though my body is asking me to keep pushing it this way – to rise above my natural tendency to hold back or go that bit easy on myself. Why should I hold back just because I am getting older? I am lucky right now not to have any physical injuries or health conditions that would prevent me from doing this running that I love, so why hold back?

Over the past year my physique has continued to change. When I first started running in 2006, I was a twelve-and-a-half stone mother of four children under the age of six. Gradually I reduced to a ten-stone woman, whose children now range in age from nine down to five. In the five years since I got my body back after having babies, I have been able to change it in ways that make me feel good about myself. My weight is no longer an issue. It's pretty stable and I am very happy to keep it that way. I still enjoy good food and when I go out socially, I never aim to hold back. But I also balance my diet with exercise. If I eat too much it means longer workouts or cutting back for a few days.

For me, this is about looking after my body and my health as well as I can on a regular basis. I generally eat well and am pretty healthy. The exercise I take gives me an appetite for good, nutritious food and I find that because my body is pushed to its physical limits, it craves a healthy overall lifestyle.

The big pay-off from pushing myself so hard physically is that I feel fantastic most of the time. My energy levels usually soar after my workout and I'm buzzing with life and energy most days. My creativity, which I love to cultivate, is in full flow.

All this makes me feel invincible and full of purpose. I'm still not sure exactly what it is I am here to do on this earth or what goals I have yet to fulfil in my life but none of that matters. What I am clear about is that I am going the right way about things – pushing my body to its limits. Even on off-days, which still come around every now and again, having this wonderful assurance keeps me grounded. Any difficulties that arise in my life are easier to cope with when my body feels fit.

Of course I do accept that I am getting older, especially on those mornings when all I feel is creak, creak, creak! But I am living in an era in which average life expectancy has risen for both men and women, with my gender now having average life spans of eighty-five years. One in ten of us, apparently, may even live to be more than a hundred. That's a lot of years to get through – and I'm not even at the half-way stage.

Right now I want to live my life with physical fitness playing a major role. In the two years since I started running, I know I have built up physical endurance that I never had before and that I can improve further. I am happy with the progress I have made so far and see opportunity for further improvement.

To any of you out there who are wondering whether exercise is really for you, or whether you were 'made' to be sporty, my advice would be: just go for it. Make a decision to do more exercise, for the sake of your health and emotional wellbeing. Getting active will leave you feeling better, happier and more connected to life. It will encourage you to look at other aspects of your world – your work, your family, your diet. It will motivate you to make positive changes all round, which in the long term will benefit not only you but everyone around you.

The medical profession has long supported the notion of an active lifestyle and it is clear to most of us by now that exercise can enhance our quality of life. Here in Ireland there are many success stories to marvel at; often what keeps these driven people on top of their game is exercise. Successful people, many of whom are in the public eye, also confess that the physical aspect of maintaining a 'body beautiful' is of utmost importance to them. They may be fortunate enough to be able to employ a personal trainer to put them through their paces and keep them motivated to do just that.

Making time for exercise, working out, running, weight-training, swimming, boxing or whatever sport tickles your fancy is a positive investment. The more you invest, the greater the return. The more physically fit you become, the more energy and drive you will have to pursue your life goals. All it takes is between half an hour and an hour each day. For anyone serious about becoming successful, that's really not an awful lot to ask.

Taking it up a level – for those who really like to push themselves in their workouts – often leads to a honing of the body that other people immediately notice. The fact that keeping fit can help you to achieve a beautiful physique is a wonderful bonus. Feeling good about our bodies is something we all aspire to. When your physical presence changes radically for the better, this makes a phenomenal statement to anyone who looks at you about just how primed for work and action your body is. A worked-out body suggests a focused mind.

Whatever line of work you are in, people will soon deduce that you mean business. There is no room for dilly-dallying. You are a serious piece of kit. Watch out!

Just knowing you feel great and fit is a powerful resource in itself. You may even play down your fitness so as not to intimidate others!

Many fitness fanatics also reveal that they use exercise as a tool to keep them grounded mentally. Allotting time for regular workouts helps them to cope with the demands people make on them and with the chaos that sometimes occurs in their lives. We meet some of these inspiring individuals here in this book.

1

Celebrity Fitness Devotees

GARY RHODES

British chef Gary Rhodes is a famous example of the 'fit for success' theory. On record for getting up religiously at 4.30 every morning to work out with weights in his private gym for forty-five minutes, the five-time Michelin star chef is an international restaurateur (including the D7 in Dublin). He is also a TV personality whose star continues to rise, most recently as a competitor on the hugely popular TV hit series *Strictly Come Dancing*. The clean-living chef describes his dedication to fitness as his 'drug'.

Gary Rhodes openly attributes his continuing success to his disciplined fitness regime and has vowed to keep working out in his basement gym as he gets older. He told *Men's Health Magazine* in 2008 that being fit makes him feel good and positive about life, in contrast to his previous tendency to feel 'worn out' after each working day.

This inspiring chef and restaurateur now has eight restaurants on the go and dozens of new projects in the pipeline. As he continues to invest time and effort into his fitness regime with punishing weights, push-ups and resistance exercises, his drive to succeed remains as strong as ever.

BILL CULLEN

One prominent Irish person who attests to using exercise to stay successful is entrepreneur and former Renault supremo Bill Cullen. This front-man for the Irish version of *The Apprentice* TV show swears by getting up early every morning to do a forty-five-minute workout, which he says fills him with energy for the rest of the day: 'I go out like a tiger after that.'

It should be pointed out that Bill Cullen is somewhat exceptional with regard to how little sleep he survives on and consequently a challenging role model for mere mortals. While Gary Rhodes gets up at 4.30 to do his workouts, Cullen gets out of bed at 4 o'clock to do his!

He doesn't go to bed particularly early either, doing a Margaret Thatcher on it by hitting the sack between 11.30 pm and midnight and working twenty-hour days seven days a week. According to Cullen, his mother had a similar routine, to all intents and purposes getting her sleep for just three to four hours in the rocking chair every night, often with a child or two in her arms. Cullen is definitely a hard act to follow but a terrific example of Irish entrepreneurial spirit.

PRESIDENT BARACK OBAMA

The new American President, Barack Obama, is another fantastic role model for fitness and success. Indeed, one of the first moves of this inspiring politician on becoming President-elect was to go for a workout. A keen basketball player, he has since designed a new gym for the White House.

In the meantime, as well as announcing that the family was to get a puppy to join them in their new home, President Obama welcomed his mother-in-law to the White House as part of the First Family. The new President's mother-in-law isn't just any ordinary granny: she is a champion sprint athlete for her age category in the US.

Go granny go!

Finding time for daily exercise is something President Obama continues to fit into his now hectic schedule – proving that if he can manage to keep fit while running the most powerful nation in the world, anyone can.

GEORGE W. BUSH

Former American President, George W. Bush, is another long-time fitness fanatic who, somewhat controversially, told US magazine *Runner's World* back in 2002 that his running track times improved after he declared war on Iraq!

He said that developing a passion for running had helped him to conquer earlier addictions to cigarettes and alcohol. Espousing exercise as crucial for the health of the nation, the former president also repeatedly highlighted the benefits of working out the body in relation to ageing. He would make no concessions: 'If I can make time for it, then anyone can,' he said.

The then President even launched an appeal to corporate America to implement work strategies with 'flexitime for exercise', as it had done with 'flexitime for families'.

President Bush counted himself among the ranks of busy people who make the effort to fit in a workout every day. He liked to get to work before 7 am and scheduled time for a run no matter what.

Every hotel room he stayed in had to have a treadmill and he even had one installed on the presidential jet, Air Force One, which allowed him to jog his way through long flights as he travelled from one country to another!

In his role as President, George W. Bush said it was his duty to set an example. Showing that he was serious about exercise sent out the message that other people should be serious too.

A one-time marathon runner, Bush added that running was a very personal thing and something he took seriously and went at 'hard'. He missed not being able to go running for as long as he liked while in office, which he said was 'one of the saddest things about the Presidency'.

At least now he is free to run as far and for as long as he wants!

CONDOLEEZZA RICE

A number of top-level American politicians are also on record as using intense fitness regimes to keep them productive in their work. Some of them might be good role models for Irish politicians.

For example, outgoing Secretary of State, Condoleezza Rice, who is fifty-four, is one such self-confessed fitness fanatic. Like Gary Rhodes, she rises at the ungodly hour of 4.30 to start her morning workout. This woman's physical appearance suggests, 'Don't mess with me,' before she even opens her mouth.

Ms Rice told American magazine *Fitness* that before work each day she likes to spend almost an hour waking up fully with exercise, usually with the encouragement of her personal trainer, a former marine. She has a preference for low-impact exercises, after years of bumps and falls as an ice-skater, and generally trains on a treadmill or elliptical machine. If she can't get to the gym, she has versions of both these machines in her own mini-gym in her apartment.

Rice once worried about her weight but now finds that her workouts and a balanced diet keep her physically and mentally in tip-top shape. She also enjoys speed-walking and hill-walking, rather than running.

No matter what her schedule is or to which part of the world she may be travelling, Rice said, she will always get out of bed to work out. What keeps her going is knowing that she will feel better afterwards, even though the activity may be hard at the time. It takes her just forty-five minutes and then she is ready to go, both physically and mentally. Inspiring lady.

2

The Fit-for-Success Candidates

For the purposes of this book I decided that the people I needed to talk to should be outright fitness fanatics who lived and breathed for the regular workouts they could schedule into their working lives. I wanted hard-core lovers of cardiovascular, aerobic and resistance training, who thrived on the sheer sweat and pain necessary to complete a workout and who would never let more than a day or two go between training sessions.

The nature of fitness training, with its many demands, followed by rewards when you reach your personal goals (running marathons, completing triathlons, beating personal bests) is hugely addictive. You know that what you are doing is hard and physically draining but you also know that your body loves being made to do so much of the work it is capable of. It wants to move and keep moving.

The fact that the people I interviewed for this book are recreational keep-fit fanatics (not a contradiction in terms) allowed me the space to explore the application of fitness training to a working life.

I selected candidates from an older age-group with an explicit purpose in mind. I wanted to show that people who are much older than is the norm for professional athletes still have it in them to work their bodies to the limit. Even though they have to fit their workouts in around work, family commitments and social engagements, they can still enjoy sporting success by participating in competitive events. While it isn't essential for fitness fanatics to be involved in competitive sports at any level, it generally seems that signing up for races and events motivates people to keep working out. I really enjoyed finding out just how competitive some of these older fitness fanatics are, regularly entering marathons, triathlons and all manner of competitive events.

Many of the older participants I had admired at various running events were not there simply to complete the distance but to perform at a certain level. They all had goals – personal bests – they wanted to achieve, which meant completing the task in a faster time and more efficient manner. They wanted to be the best they could be on that particular day in their sporting calendar.

Rather than letting the body relax and decline into old age, these individuals want to push the boundaries and show that age-related physical deterioration is a complete myth. Their love of physical fitness may have hit them at a late stage in their lives – even left them regretting that they had not trained hard as youngsters – but this makes them all the more determined to make up for lost time.

Many of these inspiring individuals treat their training almost as seriously as if they were professional athletes. They look forward to their workouts, often preferring the really hard sessions. Some even wish they could genuinely be professional athletes as this would allow them to work full-time at their training

Increased longevity and improved healthcare means that more of us than ever can hope to live longer and better quality lives than previous generations and we need to take on board certain lifestyle changes to see us through. With the good old days of hard manual labour behind us and most work stations now being sedentary, it is only to be expected that physical exercise has become more contrived. If we want to keep moving our bodies, we must take the time and trouble to do so outside work hours. We can do this by going for walks, joining a gym, taking up running, golfing, swimming, mountain climbing, rowing or martial arts. All that matters is that we sign up to do something for the sake of keeping our bodies in good nick. In return, we should see health benefits.

As I discovered in my own research, older people getting involved in exercise don't always seem to take a 'lightly, lightly' approach. Of course, no matter what your age you need to exercise caution with regard to how you treat your body but it seems that older people with a clean bill of health tend not to take things any easier than younger people.

What I wanted for this book was to interview people who were:

- fitness fanatics (without being professional athletes)
- highly successful entrepreneurs or self-employed (I wanted them to be self-motivated)
- of a certain age, that is, past the sell-by date for the typical professional athlete
- – looking the part – not only did I want them to talk the talk but I wanted their well-toned bodies to tell the story

I quickly discovered that the proof was really in the pudding. All the candidates were driven, focused, very busy people. They looked powerful, carried themselves with great dignity and seemed to glow with an inner confidence that clearly came from loving their own lifestyles.

Part of the joy of writing a book like this is getting the opportunity to meet the people who feature in it. Not all successful business people will agree to be interviewed by a journalist, as press coverage of their personal lives is often the last thing they want. But when it comes to fitness and the different ways it can be achieved, those who understand the sheer pleasure to be derived from hard workouts are usually only too happy to talk to anyone with an understanding, listening ear. That's because this fitness business is more than a hobby to those who invest time in it – it is an absolute passion, something they do that may cause discomfort at the time but which has a positive payback in other aspects of their lives.

It was especially rewarding to meet fitness fanatics in the flesh and find them exactly as I expected them to be. Even if some of them claimed that they were not obsessed by fitness, merely healthily addicted to their preferred sport or workout routines, it was evident to me that – allowing for their work, their families and other important aspects of their lives – they were indeed obsessed – and loving it!

They spent time figuring out exactly when and how they would fit in their next workout: considering whether it should be a hell-for-leather, flat-out session, a mid-tempo recovery workout, or perhaps just a filler – a stretch and warm-down to keep the muscles ticking over until the next big one.

Anyone who loves exercise admits – to themselves at

– that the buzz from working out can't be beaten. So why would anyone who knows this ever want to give it up? All that matters is that the body is challenged by aerobic, cardiovascular and/or resistance/weight-bearing exercise on an ongoing basis. While exercise sessions may be physically demanding, the feel-good reward afterwards is such that every moment of suffering seems worthwhile. Anyone who doesn't know just how good a workout can leave you feeling – especially after it's over – doesn't know what they're missing.

3

Dr Mick Loftus

Dr Mick Loftus, 79, has been a general practitioner in his hometown of Crossmolina, County Mayo, for more than forty years and is involved in numerous community and national organisations. The former coroner for north Mayo and relentless campaigner against the association of alcohol with sport represented his home county in senior and junior All-Irelands in the 1940s and 1950s, going on to referee two All-Ireland finals before serving for three terms as President of the GAA during the 1980s.

Dr Loftus was busy with administrative work and a thriving medical practice in his middle years, and physical fitness slipped from his life during that period. Weighing in at fifteen stone on his sixtieth birthday, he vowed to become physically fit once more and took up walking After a while his walks turned into runs and by the age of seventy-eight, Dr Loftus had progressed to a fitness regime that included a three-quarter-hour run every night. Since then, Dr Loftus, who is approaching his eightieth birthday, has upped the ante to take in four miles on his nightly run. Indeed, he now plans to mark his milestone birthday by running his first marathon in 2009.

In 2006, Dr Loftus won gold in the 3000-metre race at the World Senior Games in Utah, US, as well as three silver medals in the 8000, 1500 and 5000-metre races. He received a hero's welcome on his return home to Crossmolina. His many personal, community and sporting achievements have been recognised on national and international stages throughout his lifetime.

Dr Mick believes that exercise is crucial to health and even more important as we get older. He brooks no argument that age is a barrier to exercise, insisting instead that the older people get, the more exercise they should be doing. In *Anyone Can Run*, Dr Mick declared his intention of exercising hard for the rest of his life. For the purposes of *Fit for Success* I decided to check up on him as his eightieth birthday approaches to see if he is sticking to his resolve.

So, Dr Mick, you're still running?

'I'm still running, yes. I do it most nights. Of course the time has changed for winter but I still go out in the dark and the moon lights up the road. If it's a very bad night I might do a quarter of an hour on the treadmill.

'I do a four-mile loop now instead of my usual three. The three-miler took a route through the town but now the 'mad doc' is going round the back by another road instead, doing a U-shaped run.

'It wasn't intentional that I increased distance, just that it kept me out of the town and people having to see me go. Coming to my age I mightn't be able to do it as well as I could but I still go at it-non stop and would be back in around forty-five to fifty minutes.'

How long does Dr Mick see himself running like this?

'I maintain I will keep going indefinitely. I look forward

to my run every night and on a Sunday after Mass, Edie and I go down to Enniscrone, a beautiful beach, and while I jog, she walks.

'During the week I work in the surgery. At 8.15 I open up, go through a few letters, out to Mass, a cup of tea at the house, back here by ten at the latest and working through to 1.30 pm, depending on who's looking for me. Then I'm back again at 2.45 pm, through to 5.30 pm.

'Tonight, believe it or not, I'm going to my computer course as well. I've signed up for a twelve-week two-hour class to learn a whole lot of things about computers from the basics up. I can use the computer to prepare things and make appointments but it always annoyed me that I couldn't do it properly so I decided on the course. I do find it fairly taxing after being here all day as you need to concentrate on it but I really want to master the thing.

'In the evening, after I've read the papers, I may do a bit of work until I hit the hay at 11.30. No sooner am I there than I'm asleep. I've never had to take a sleeping tablet in my life. People feel as you get older you have to take them but I've never subscribed to that. I think the whole reason for my sleeping so well is the exercise.'

Although a late convert to regular exercise, Dr Mick had a certain amount of activity over the years that must have helped him later on.

'I did keep some notes from years back of what I was doing from an exercise point of view. During my presidency of the GAA, for instance, I see I did a bit of running. I've one note here of a run across Sydney Harbour Bridge and another over the Golden Gate Bridge in San Francisco. So it's good to see I took some advantage of the travel involved.

'All the same, that was around the time my weight hit a high of fifteen stone five pounds. Despite the running there were always the dinners. But I never went on a diet. I just cut down gradually on the food without going off anything in particular. The result was I took off almost three stone, primarily through exercise, avoiding all fatty foods and eating more fruit. I'm not looking at everything I eat but I am very careful and take no second helpings.'

Getting older has never been a problem for Dr Mick and even his eightieth birthday, around the corner, is just another number.

'As you age you can take on more and more exercise. I never think I'm old. I laugh when I think I'm talking now and I'm eighty. I never think of death. I attribute it all to the exercise and to being involved in so many things. If I have to go eventually, I think I'd like to be shot.'

Dr Mick never considered retiring from his work when he hit official pension age – or indeed at any time after that.

'Retiring at sixty-five is conditioning people to think, "I'm not up to it any longer." Socially and physiologically they think it's normal to start really ageing then but people should get away from this idea that it's normal to stop doing things they've always done. It's not normal. People should be involved and stay involved. Maybe it's good that I am this way. So many patients ask me how I do it so at least they see it can be done.

'The reality is that people are ageist. Younger people are certainly ageist but we elderly are more ageist than anybody else. People say, "Oh I'm this age, why should I be in the pool swimming? That's not the place for me. You have to act your age." Or else they say they have a pain in their knee or their back so they can't do anything. It's just an excuse, even though they all appreciate and understand that exercise is good. But they just make the decision that it's not for them.'

Working to change people's minds about this is the most difficult part, according to Dr Mick.

'The question is how to motivate them. The furore over the threatened medical card withdrawal in the budget got 10,000 pensioners out marching. The next day, if you said to them will you go for a walk, 80% of them wouldn't have budged. They would have said they couldn't go out the door because it was raining. And sure it rained like hell the day of the march! The difference was that they were motivated to take action on the march because it was the money that motivated them. If only we had something else to motivate them and keep them motivated.'

Unfortunately, that is a big ask, as Dr Mick knows well from his fifty years' experience as a GP.

'Talking to elderly patients you find that's just the way they think: that they shouldn't be out except maybe for taking a walk. When I say then they should be walking fairly fast to get the heart going, they take no heed. So what many of them are doing is just having a stroll and that gets them out in the fresh air but it won't give them the real benefits that come from proper exercise.'

Dr Mick also believes that the ageist influence of older people on their peers is detrimental.

'Older people tell one another to act their age. The standard message is: you're no good after sixty-five, once you retire. Retirement has this effect: people thinking they should sit down, put the feet up, maybe do a bit of gardening. I know some get into golf and fair dues to them for that – but I don't know if golf has the same health benefits as running.

'When people are less active they're sitting around and then they're inclined to eat more so obesity is another issue as we get older. Look around anywhere, even at people in middle age. You see players who were top footballers or who were very active up to maybe forty years of age. They give up their exercise and next thing, they're obese.

'Or look at the farmers, who have gone from fit and lean to heavy people operating machinery. It's a big change. They used to be thin from all the labour that was involved in their work – having to harrow, plough, use the spade. Now the tractors and machines do practically everything. I'd say in a lot of cases they could leave their tractors behind them and go walking!

'Age is no barrier to exercise and should not be regarded as such. Maybe progress is more difficult, although the majority of older people who exercise agree that exercise keeps them healthy. But our current situation is that older people are the least active generation, despite the findings of the World Health Organisation and various research studies that show that there is considerable potential for prevention of heart disease in older people if they participate in sport and competition. Indeed, the health-enhancing benefits of exercise relate particularly to the older group, according to the WHO.'

As a competing 'senior' runner himself, Dr Mick has grown accustomed to racing against his peers.

'I haven't cut back at all just because I'm getting on. When I go over to compete in the World Masters' Championships in St George, Utah, everyone there is over fifty-five. There are 10,000 of us from all over the world. One man over eighty had cancer in the kidney but you would never know it to see him running around. It's a day like that we should be having here in Ireland, just to show people what can be done.'

The notion of running his first marathon has become more appealing to Dr Mick over time.

'I had it in the back of my head to do the marathon in Dublin last year but I hadn't prepared properly for it. But now I am doing longer runs than usual and I'm thinking of a few new routes to give me extra miles. Of course it would be a case of jogging and walking as I see fit but that would be fine. I've one loop in mind now that would give me twenty-one miles. I did a twelve-miler there not so long ago as a fundraiser and didn't have any problems. That took me two-and-a-half hours so I'm looking at over five hours for a marathon and I would be happy with that.

'None of us can achieve what we see the Africans and Russians and the Paula Radcliffes of this world doing but I still think it's out there for the ordinary people. The way I started, after having been retired from football for years, was by going out walking. I would then do thirty to forty yards jogging, then walk again, gradually increasing the distances over time. People say they can't find the time to do this but I see them going out to dinner regularly and they can make the time for that. So, you know, you can always make the time for exercise – and all it takes is thirty minutes a day.

'If we could just get the fifty to sixty age-group to start taking exercise, the financial and social benefits to the state and the health system would be immense. The day after the presidential election in America we saw Barack Obama come out of the gym. He looks the part too. Unfortunately we've no such role models among our political leaders.'

Dr Mick is keen to remind people of the many health benefits that accrue from fitness.

'Physiologically, the biggest benefit is to the cardiovascular system, which governs blood pressure and contributes to the prevention of strokes and heart attacks. This is an immense help. Next there are the benefits to the alimentary system. For people who sit around a lot, constipation is often an issue. Exercise is very good in relation to this as it gets the system moving and working as it should. Regular exercise has also been shown to slow down the onset of Alzheimer's, reversing brain decline. Aerobic exercise can reverse age decline and obesity and basically exercise can play a role in all health issues. I see of late that they are even talking about the benefits exercise can have in preventing breast cancer.

'So the health benefits that come from exercise can affect every aspect of your life. Exercise reawakens the whole body energy. It doesn't have to be running. Any exercise can have the same effect.'

Dr Mick attributes his own happy disposition to the fact that he works out so much.

'You feel far better even getting up in the morning. I wake up at 7.15, listen to the news and then I'm up. Attending all the meetings I have to go to, even at my age, is something I just never think about because of the way I feel.

'I also find my attitude to people is always balanced. I never lose the cool with them. I think it's all because I feel good, so I wouldn't be complaining. People ask how I can still concentrate at my age. I find I can concentrate away and when I come back from the evening run, I feel like a two-year old. I could tackle into another day's work!

'I'd say my productivity at the moment is as good as the

day I started working here. I think your attitude remains very good when you're fit. You don't mind tackling anything. Naturally some things take a lot out of you but once you're fit, you can tackle them. If you have worries, exercise can help that too. There are just so many positives. You go to bed, you're asleep – no problems there. I often have to get up for the train at 5.30 in the morning. That's no problem either and I'll always be well rested. I do my day in Dublin, I don't take the Luas but walk in from the station if I have time and walk back to the station because I miss my runs on those days. One thing I can't do yet is run with the suit on!

'Naturally in the profession I'm in, I'm dealing with life and death issues and it is important that I make the right decisions. Being fit helps me to address that area. Of course I am anxious to do the right thing by my patients. I can give people more attention because I have the energy to do so.

'I think the brain is more active as a result of exercise, as we see from all the studies. Fit people are better able to tackle situations. We have to try hard to get the message across that exercise brings real benefits in every area of your life. I can't see any area of life that it doesn't improve. I'm as busy as anyone. Yesterday I had to be in Castlebar for work, the day before that I was in Dublin but I can still make the time for exercise.

'When I look back over the years, what I wanted was to have my practice at the top of the ladder. I had to give it time, energy and commitment to achieve that and that is what I have been able to do as a result of keeping fit.'

Scheduling a daily four-mile run isn't excessive, according to Dr Mick.

'I'm not hung up on exercise. I just do it. If I miss a night, fair enough. But I'd find if I missed two nights or so I would be getting keen to go.

'I often sit there in the surgery, looking forward to the run in the evening. Now it was hard last weekend because when I looked out the window the weather did look awful but when I was out in the shorts and T-shirt, it was not too bad. A lady once asked me did I not get cold in the legs but I don't even think about it. I find the sleeveless jacket thing great.

'I do think there are more people out running now. I suppose I make some of them feel guilty. If I was in my fifties people probably wouldn't take as much notice.

'I should have taken up running earlier but my exercise was centred around training for football and then dropping out around forty. That's the typical football era. But the benefits that would accrue in later life, not only to the individual but also to society, if we could keep our training going after forty, would be immense.

'I even feel in regard to the alcohol problem in this country that if people were fit, they wouldn't be as inclined to drink or smoke. There wouldn't be this thing of them just going to games, watching others playing, going to the pub and then having a big meal. Just to get away from that would be so good.'

Dr Mick regrets taking that typical pause from exercise after he stopped playing competitive football.

'I definitely would have run a marathon or two if I had got into this sooner. I'll have to have a go at it some time. I know I have a Pacemaker but that never occurs to me. The old knee is my only trouble as I have arthritis from a bad football injury I got long ago. But I just wonder if I could do the twenty-six miles and that's what I'm hoping to find out. A new knee would be the ideal – maybe next year. *Le cúnamh Dé.*

4

James Murphy

As well as building up his hugely successful healthcare, beauty and lifestyle products company, Lifes2good and performing regular gigs as one of the Galway Tenors, Athenry native and family man James Murphy happens to be a keen triathlon participant.

James came to triathlons for the first time only when he entered his forties. He is now forty-seven and totally hooked. In the intervening years, the triathlon has become the fastest-growing individual sport in the world, with droves of young and old training for events.

James's company, Lifes2good, started life as Irish Response Limited in 1997, distributing health and beauty products. Over the years, with product endorsements from well-known people including golfer Christy O'Connor, Amanda Brunker, Glenda Gilsen, Keith Wood, and UK celebrities Cheryl Baker, Lee Sharpe, Virginia Wade and Jenny Bond, the company developed a number of brand leaders. Categories include skincare and pain-relief products. Some of the leading sellers include Viviscal, Magnetic Therapy, the Slender range of weight-loss supplements, Pu'erh Tea, YSX cosmetics treatments and Vivida anti-ageing supplements and creams.

Last year, 2008, saw particularly strong growth by the company, which scooped a €5 million-distribution deal for Lifes2good products in Brazil and a second deal worth up to €10 million in Beijing. This involved the launch of the company's Vivida anti-ageing food supplement in the Chinese market.

Aiming for nothing short of saturation, James commented at the time that the company would be focusing on 'affluent females in Beijing – with a target market of fifty million'. He also declared his intention of launching other Lifes2good products in the Chinese market.

James added: 'Lifes2good is about providing proven products that fit easily into people's lifestyles. It has taken some years to narrow down the niche problem areas where modern lifestyles make it difficult for people to stay on top. Most of our time and money has been spent developing drug-free alternatives for those serious concerns.'

A dynamic company enjoying rapid and substantial growth, Lifes2good is now recognised by both the industry it serves and consumers as a quality organisation promoting highly innovative, effective, natural product brands.

Making time for fitness and exercise has always been a priority for James, but he waited until he was possibly at his busiest forging a career as an entrepreneur before deciding to have a go at his first triathlon.

'In college I played hurling and handball, then got into rugby but I always did a bit of cross-country and long distance running, just to keep in shape. Over time I got more into rugby and running short distances.

'You know how it is then when you settle down and start having kids. You hit your thirties and forget about exercise.

So there's no training. I see it all the time now. Young fellows with beer bellies, working really hard, travelling. They find it impossible to train because they just don't have the energy.

'Next thing you're hitting forty, the kids are grown up and your energy levels start to come back as you don't have to get up at night. All you need then is a trigger and I got mine when I sponsored the first triathlon in Galway back in 2001. I met all the participants, found they were such a fine bunch of people and said, to hell with this, I'd better get stuck in myself. So I started training and did my first triathlon that first year.'

It wasn't simply a case of going from zero to a hundred overnight, as James discovered that building up his capacity for the three core triathlon disciplines of swimming, running and cycling required dedicated training.

'I found it incredibly tough. You really need to train for two years to get into triathlons. The first season you just about get there. The body has to adapt. I hadn't done swimming or cycling before. At the beginning my times were around three and a half hours. That didn't put me off. Once I got into the habit of the training, I really liked it. You get such a kick being able to swim the distance. It's a real buzz and it keeps you at it and at it.

'Swimming in the pool is easy enough. Sixty lengths sounds hard but it's actually OK. It only takes half an hour to get up to 1500 metres. I would never have been able to do that distance at the start. It was a real case of building it up.

'As far as the cycling is concerned, well, with conditions as they are in Ireland, you have to be very careful. It's often icy or wet and if you come off the bike, you're going to get badly injured.

'Some of the roads that used to be good for cycling here in Galway, such as out by Moycullen, are now so busy it's dangerous. I would often go out and back to Spiddal, covering thirty-five kilometres, or at the weekends I might go further out to the TG4 headquarters [at Indreabhán] for a sixty-four-kilometre round trip, coming back to go for my run. Or else I might run and swim and cycle one after the other, depending. But over the past year I would always do at least one of the event distances in each training session. It's easier for me now: it doesn't feel so long because I've got to that level of fitness. What you really need in the triathlon are endurance and stamina, as opposed to speed.

'I train continuously through the year and because triathlons are my sport, I will always be cross-training between the disciplines of swimming, running and riding the bike.

'The typical Olympic-standard triathlon includes a 1.5k swim, a forty-kilometre bike ride and a ten-kilometre run. These are quite some distances so you have to be doing them every single week, with at least one training session in each of the disciplines.

'So you can cover this over maybe three days a week or closer to the summer, when the triathlon calendar is in full swing, you would ultimately like to cover each discipline twice a week. So I might do two events in one day, for instance cycle, then get off the bike and run. As the date of the event moves closer, I try to train at all three disciplines in the one workout.

'Usually I ramp up my training in April and May so that I'm ready to race in the competitions in June. You're always trying to get a bit faster and for me, swimming is the activity that holds me back. I would have been able to swim only about twenty-five metres up to the age of forty. My son, Neil, got me doing more after I trained with him. I just kept swimming and found that the more you train, the more you can do. It's like anything.

'The great thing about all this training is that it keeps me in great shape. In the middle of the season I'm incredibly slim, which for me is 77-82kg. That's my perfect weight when I wouldn't have a pick on me. I can drink as many pints and eat as many biscuits as I like. That's the problem with getting older. You're not burning the calories off so you cannot get the weight down unless you eat less. Also, there's a lot of calories in alcohol and in Ireland we like to drink. I'm amazed we don't have even more obese people.'

James also makes sure to fit in time to train on his many business trips abroad.

'I travel quite a bit but I just build my training into it. I make sure there is a pool or at least a gym in the hotel, or that I am close to a park. Next week, for instance, I'll be in Hong Kong and Korea. I've checked that both hotels I'm staying in have the training facilities I need.'

Getting older is having a positive effect on James's performance: his triathlon times have been improving with his growing fitness.

'I did the Olympic Triathlon in Chicago last year in a time of two hours thirty-seven. That was unbelievable for me because usually if I get around in three hours I'm happy. The weather is much calmer in the US so you get a better swim and it's so well organised too. The roads are flat so you're able to go like the clappers. I did one hour eight minutes on the bike – against my best of one hour fifteen at the time. The transition times also worked quickly for me.

'The Chicago Triathlon started at 9 am and had 8,000 competitors. The weather was very warm. There's a lot of science in triathlons. You're constantly looking for things to boost your performance and you need to watch your salt and sugar intake.

'It's the fastest-growing sport in the world and there are many products now as well as specific gear. It's an Olympic sport and an incredible one. You have the usual contingent of competitors every year and many new people keep coming in.

'In the swim, you usually have to go out as far as two buoys in the water but often you can't see anything, which is a bit of a nuisance. You're in such a trough with the waves, all you can see is guys going all over the place. So you're just hell-bent on getting the swim done as quickly as possible, although some people like to pace themselves. But I go like hell because I think it's great and there's no point holding back your energy to sprint the last kilometre. You have to push yourself hard if you want to get the times.

'There are two triathlons I do in Sweden in the summer and it's fabulous over there. They're so well organised. They close down the town, as they do for the Athlone Triathlon. You get a great buzz with the people along the routes, because normally you're by yourself.

'Numbers are capped at all events and people are graded according to their age categories. Overall the triathlon is a very nice social event and the euphoria when you've done one is great. It's all about people getting to know each other, people staying over together. It's a great challenge for people who are interested in sport but who don't want to race or be so competitive that it's all about winning. The beauty of the triathlon is that you're always picking off people, although I wouldn't get carried away with the times.'

James now likes to do at least five triathlons in Ireland each summer and others abroad. 'Once you get yourself into peak condition you could do them every week and there is such a mixture of sprint and full triathlons events on all the time that it's great.

'The sport most people are afraid of is the swim. You see a lot of people getting stranded in the water. They are very slow, perhaps not doing the front crawl but the breast stroke. They get into trouble but at least they have wetsuits on and that keeps them safe.

'I swam once in a gale-force 5 wind. You're getting badly beaten by the waves but because of the wetsuit – which is obligatory – you're not going to sink. You may take in gulps of water and panic but you're not going to go down.'

Training in deep sea waters can be scary too. 'When you're out on your own, you could run into a dolphin and be just as afraid of that as if you met a shark. There are loads of jellyfish to wade through. But you have to train in the sea because that's where the race will be. Sometimes I swim in the Corrib as well. The reality is, once you stick on the wetsuit, you can swim anywhere.'

Irish sea creatures may be scary when you meet them during your swimming training, but in America there are worse hazards: 'They have a triathlon out in San Diego [California] and there are sharks in the waters there. I was over there a month ago and went for a run. The sharks actually come into the bay. There's another swim across to Alcatraz and the bastards come in there too!'

James is happy sticking with triathlons and isn't a fan of

marathon-running or 'super triathlons' such as the Iron Man.

'The Iron Man is an event that entails a 3.8-kilometre swim, a 200-kilometre bike ride and a marathon but I have no interest in that. I've never done a marathon and don't want to either, although I have raced half-marathons. You have to understand the damage you can do to your body when you do that kind of distance. Your body will say you can do it but if your body isn't right, you will know all about it later.

'It's not that I'm against doing marathons altogether but it's just such a long time to be running. Then there's all that talk about hitting the wall, when your body wants to give up. If you want to do something that keeps you going that long and gives you the buzz you're looking for, I recommend triathlon, where you're doing the three disciplines and building up confidence in each.'

And the worst thing about triathlons?

'The worst thing about triathlons is that they can be called off! The Vancouver event was called off this year because the water was too cold.'

So what's a typical day's training?

'At the moment I would be doing a minimum of five days and on average six training days a week. I get up at 7 am, do an hour's training and get into work for 9.30. I don't like going on the bike in the morning because there is just too much traffic and motorists have no respect for bikes. Cars come close and buses come even closer and they have no clue how dangerous that is. If you're hit, you're gone, simple as that.

'I've come off the bike a few times. Once I had a big skid, wearing just my shorts. I left skin on the road. A lot of guys break their collarbones.'

James wasn't sure how his body felt when his fortieth birthday came along: 'In 2001, when I got to forty, I looked in the mirror and asked myself: what will it be like from here? I didn't like what I saw and decided I needed some new stimulation in my life, some challenge. At that time I felt I really wanted to make a serious success of something. I wanted to make a hell of a lot of money and then move on to the next thing.

'In 1991 I came back from Brussels, where I had been living, to start Slendertone for this guy and came up with a strategy to make it a success. In 1997 I got out of it because I wanted to start up and work for myself. That was when Lifes2good came into existence.

'As you get older you become even more focused. Now I know I don't want to have a business that is just providing an income or a lifestyle. A lot of people are in that trap of falling in love with a business and wanting to keep at it but they may not be as productive or as focused on the bottom line as they could be. They just end up living for the business.

'This company of mine, Lifes2good, is an international business with great brands. I want to sell it and move on, so for me it's a case of needing to have a package in place and objectives that have to be met, rather than just running it as a "Let's wait and see how things are in a few years' time." Within three to five years I will have packaged and sold this business. I believe a lot of businesses could be much more productive if their owners were focused on building up the businesses and moving on to something else.'

James credits much of his ability to focus so clearly to his ongoing fitness regime.

'It helps me with my business in terms of my energy levels.

I travel a lot and work long and hard but I'm not a workaholic. I don't work at weekends and I try to get out at a reasonable hour each day but if something is up I do try to get it done. When I'm travelling I work. I never take a few extra days to see a place. It's just do the work and get out.

'The training gives me tremendous discipline. Often, when people travel abroad for work a lot, they suffer with jet-lag and tiredness. Then they get there and because of how they feel, they might take a drink or over-indulge in food. Then they end up not having any energy and it's a vicious circle. They are like crocks, only performing at 60% of their potential and suffering from loss of concentration.

'But if you have discipline and you're going to bed at a good time and getting up fresh, you're fine. When I get across to Korea, after a sleep the first thing I do is work out. This will get the jet-lag out of the system and I will be much more productive. I train and because of that I sleep properly. When I'm travelling to the United States I tend to sleep quickly. I force myself to sleep and training helps to get you physically tired.

'There's no question that the fitter you are the more focused and alert you are. So you're much more productive. You're thinking about getting the work done so that you can train and get your times. I travel somewhere most weeks so I have to get a lot of work handled when I am here but because I'm fit I have more energy to do all that.'

Being one of the Galway Tenors is another great love in James's life. Indeed, if he can achieve his business model he may be able to dedicate himself to operatic singing.

'I perform with two others, one professional – Frank Naughton – and one semi-professional, Sean Costello. I have a good voice but the problem is that I don't train it. I would love to be able to do more performing and bigger gigs if possible. For example we did a corporate gig for 5000 people over three nights at the K Club this year and we also sang during the Ryder Cup. We sing each year at the Oyster Festival in Galway and we do a number of charity events. We're a bit different and that's why people like us. We like to have a laugh with it.'

Taking up sport in his forties has not only concentrated James's business mind but made his thoughts about life in general more philosophical.

'Sport is a great tool. The body needs it because we do so much less physical work than our grandparents and parents. Our generation is not getting any exercise from work. If we don't supplement with exercise we're going to get more unhealthy for sure. No doubt people won't live as long. There will be ferocious pressure in healthcare when people in their sixties and seventies won't be as healthy. This will cost the state a fortune.

'The way I look at life is this: if you look at the first twenty years, that's about getting your body to reach its full growth. You spend most of that time just trying to learn.

'Over the next twenty years it's all about trying to get some wealth, assets, a lifestyle – deciding what you want to do with your life.

'Then at forty you realise, Jesus, I'm forty! You have to start thinking about putting money away, a pension, thinking about the kids getting older

'Then you get to sixty and at sixty the problem is you're going to have another twenty years. If you haven't looked after yourself between forty and sixty, you're going to have an awful time between sixty and eighty. People won't be looking forward to it.

'But you can put in the good work in advance so that at forty, you know you've lived only half your life and you can look forward to enjoying the rest. Whether you like it or not you're going to live a lot longer, so in your forties you have to decide how you want to live the rest of your life.

'My advice would be to find something that will stimulate you and train for it. It doesn't matter whether you were ever into sport before. You can start at any time.

'People don't understand what they're going to be like when they're in their sixties. I think that if I'm enjoying life then as much as I am now, in my forties, I will just want it to continue. I want to be able to have the craic in my sixties and the idea of going out to grass at that age is just daft.

'Even in your seventies you can do triathlons. One of the things that impressed me the most when I did the Galway Triathlon was a seventy-two year old man who did it in four hours. This means you can be in good condition into your eighties and then that brings you up to your nineties and so on, up to a hundred. If you can exercise all the way up to eighty, eighty to a hundred might not be too bad.'

Exercising for the good of your health is one thing but the satisfaction is even greater when you know your lifestyle is also having a positive impact on the younger generation.

'My competing in events like triathlon at my age is great for the kids: they are really impressed by it. In fact, the number of people who tell me they are seriously impressed by what I do confirms that I am right to be doing this. If they in turn were stimulated to do the same thing that would be terrific. I'm a great believer in leading by example.'

James is married to Maria and the couple have three boys and one girl, aged seventeen, sixteen, thirteen and eleven. Has his influence rubbed off enough to get them involved in triathlons?

'Well, I didn't get Maria into it as much as myself but she does swim every day with a bunch of girls and we also have a cocker spaniel that needs lots of exercise! Our eldest fellow is in the Connaught Academy for rugby, the next fellow is big into wind-surfing, hurling and rugby, our daughter is on the under-16 Irish hockey panel and the youngest plays tennis and golf and is rugby-mad. I'd like to think we had an influence on that because they're seeing us not only in good shape but active.'

What happens if James ever misses a day of training or becomes ill?

'It's inevitable that you will sometimes have a cold or some bug or other and you have to rest. But my recovery times have improved with my fitness. If I miss two days of training in a row I go mad. My wife will say, "Let's just organise to get him into a pool." You've built up a lot of stamina and endurance and it's the adrenaline you're looking to get back.'

In the winter, when triathlon events are few and far-between, James just keeps tipping away at his training. 'I'd love to think that in a couple of years, when I have time, I could just go on a circuit of triathlons around the world. I would enter events in different countries, build up my training and drive around seeing things. I know that when we got married, Maria didn't bargain for all the time I spend training but it's very good for health and your health is your wealth.'

5

Ray O'Connor

Ray O'Connor established Proactive – one of Galway's most successful design and marketing companies – in 1995 at the age of twenty-five. Today the company employs a staff of eighteen, with Ray overseeing design projects as Creative Director.

During the early years of Proactive, while the company was going through a steep growing curve, Ray discovered marathon-running. In 2008 he ran ten marathons in ten days as part of the famous May Brathay Challenge in the UK. To date, Ray has run a total of fifty-three marathons and has now set himself the task of completing a hundred by 2012 – which will entitle him to membership of the 100 Marathon Club, something he has long coveted.

Having to find time for the running he so loves has helped Ray to become more relaxed, more disciplined, more organised and more successful in his career. He attributes his continuing productivity to his running achievements and is convinced that when he himself is at peak fitness his business also performs at its best.

Just because he could go out the door at the drop of a hat and run twenty-six miles doesn't mean that Ray considers himself super-fit. In fact, Ray O'Connor maintains he isn't properly fit at all at the moment and is gearing himself up for a higher standard of running during 2009.

Ray is father to Adam, aged eighteen, Aaron, aged fifteen, Alex, aged nine, and Evan, aged six. Although he describes himself as not 'very social or outgoing', Ray has acquired a certain popular reputation in his native county over the years, winning a Galway Person of the Year Award in 2008.

Ray is also the man behind the Connemara Marathon – which takes place in April each year and now attracts up to 4,000 entries from all over the world – and runireland. com, the on-line event booking and running news website. He is a motivational speaker on behalf of Croi [the West of Ireland Cardiology Foundation] and, with his tall, finely-honed physique and enthusiastic personality, is an inspiration to anyone hoping to understand the secrets of success.

Ray explains:

'I started Proactive in 1995, when I was twenty-five. I had two kids and it was fairly full-on starting a new business too. My trade as a graphic designer wasn't huge then. I was a bit of a trend-setter, I suppose. I was young.

'I was formally trained on the job, starting at the age of thirteen and continuing as an apprentice after I left school at sixteen. I was very clear what I wanted to be. I stole a march on other printers and went from printing directly into the computer age, which gave me a head start.'

The company had a strong opening market as there was an appetite for new design ideas at the time, something Ray had plenty of.

'We were completely new. The stuff I was producing was so different. The only problem – and this is one I have even now – is that everything always depended on Ray O'Connor and everyone wanted my finger on the job. It was very hard to manage getting away from that.

'I was working crazy hours, eighteen hours a day, from 7 am to 9 pm. It was very stressful and I was smoking thirty fags a day. I didn't feel unhealthy but mentally I must have been all over the place. But the business was good to us. We expanded and as the bills mounted, the stress mounted. It's a natural spiral.

'On the one hand it's nice knowing the company depends on you but on the other, when you want to go home, it isn't nice at all. Proactive has grown over the years to the point that I now have a staff of eighteen. Up to the time I ran my first marathon, we were really busy. We moved from town centre premises at Mayoralty House up here to Liosban Industrial Estate and expanded very quickly. We went from seven to fourteen staff in the space of six months. It was a big change for the business and for me. Maybe taking on a marathon was a good distraction from the negatives that go with expanding. I'm a very positive person and I've always surrounded myself with positive people. I got a great buzz out of running so, yes, it was a very positive distraction.

'With all that was going on at work I was probably looking for an outlet. I absolutely love doing what I do and I always did. Sometimes people really appreciate what I do: they tell me that what sets me apart is that I make things look good. Hearing this makes it all worthwhile. Proactive has developed into a company that helps people sell products through marketing, design and PR. Basically we cover anything to do with design and have a very diverse client portfolio, including GMIT, the NUI Tipperary Institute and some multinationals. So it's nice and diverse. If someone comes in off the street to us with a new device to sell, we'll help to bring it to the market.

'I did a lot of work for Croi and in late March 2000, the CEO, Neil Johnson, told me he was getting a team together to run the New York marathon six months later as a fund-raiser. I said I'd do it but he just laughed at me. I was actually thinner then. I've put on nearly two stone since I started running.'

Anyone meeting Ray O'Connor in the flesh might well wonder where exactly that two stone went, as he still looks as skinny as a rake!

'Putting on the weight was an interesting side-effect of the whole running thing but I probably did look unhealthy before. I was twenty-nine when I started running and I was thinking back to when I was a kid and ran with the Galway City Harriers between the ages of ten and twelve. I played hurling and soccer up to fifteen and was probably a normal fit, healthy teenager. But then when I started to work, women and drink became more important.

'The first thing I did was give up the fags. I said to myself that if I replaced them with something else I would be able to stick it out and the replacement was to be the running. Within a week, there was an article in the paper about me doing New York, as my business was being profiled at that point.

'I got it into my head that if I smoked one cigarette, that was it – I would have blown the whole thing. I remember my very first training session up to Dangan, where as a kid I often ran from my home in Newcastle a mile away. I had to do one mile – four laps – and I couldn't finish my first mile. I felt a complete failure and knew I needed to take a step back. I took the approach of running a bit and then walking a bit.

'People think it is so easy to do a mile. They see a jogger on the prom and it looks easy. Maybe it's the whole good aura they give off but the truth is, very few are running gracefully along. We're all sweating and feeling tired.'

Ray has come a long way since those first, difficult training runs.

'I think I'm beginning to enjoy running now as I'm in a different bracket. When I go out training, I train a lot on my own as I usually have a particular goal in mind. My programmes for a marathon now are just two weeks long, maybe even one week, because I do them so regularly.

'For that first marathon in New York in 2000, I built the training up to just thirteen miles. I suffered from injuries and there was a whole lot of things going on. On the day itself, I walked the first six miles. There were two girls with me who were walkers and I got it into my head that I might even walk it with them. But at mile six I felt confident enough to take off and the going went well up to the twentieth mile. In the end I finished the marathon in five hours fifteen minutes with a run-walk approach. What I did there was perfect.

'I had already entered for my second marathon. I just knew this was the thing I wanted to do, running marathons. I don't know why. I think I had the notion because when I was a kid, a friend of mine had an uncle who had run fifty-six marathons. Back in the early 1980s I was on the water station at the old Galway marathon. So I've always been sort of aware of marathon running.

'Anyway I had booked in to do the London marathon as an overseas entry. I trained a bit better for that over the following six months and finished it in four hours fifty-nine minutes. I was really elated: all I wanted was to come in under five hours. I kept telling myself, 'I'm a runner now, I did it!'

'It was unbelievable at the finish line. Seeing someone dressed as a Womble come in just behind me took a bit of the shine off it, though, as I considered myself to be a runner but he made it look as if anyone – or anything – could do it!

'People ask what I think about when I run but it's a blank, which isn't a bad thing. You're just checking yourself out, how your body feels, your mind. We don't ever do that – stop to think 'How am I?' – except maybe when we're sick and it's negative. Running is always a pleasant distraction and time out for me. I'm not a selfish person and I don't take time out otherwise to look after myself.

'I remember I was on a marathon in Longford, around my thirtieth, and going through a bad patch at the twenty-second mile. I was running alongside this girl and she knew I was feeling rough, so she talked me through each part of my body from my head to my toes, asking how each part felt: were they sore? As I answered that each part felt fine I realised that there was really nothing wrong with me. This convinced me that I was OK and I felt OK then. I always remember that.

'As the business was expanding, I was also getting more competitive about running. It was like the two were feeding off each other and were completely linked. You see that especially when you're fit. I'm not always fit in the sense that I'm on top form at peak fitness. For instance, if you asked me to go for a run this afternoon I would run twenty-six miles but I don't consider that to be fitness. I'd like to be able to run twenty-six miles more easily!

'I started to get really fit in 2001 for my third marathon, which was in Chicago. I trained hard and wanted to finish in or around four hours. It was funny. Even though I've done fifty-three marathons in total now, Chicago still stands out as the most terrifying starting line I've ever been on. I was so terrified I was white, green even. I was so nervous, even though I had trained. I was going for a time so I was racing, competing with the distance. I wanted to conquer it. I haven't been as nervous since.

'Looking back I can see that it was all self-imposed pressure. I did break down to a walk at the twenty-fifth mile and my finishing time was four hours thirteen minutes. I was disappointed but I needed to put it in perspective and remind myself that eleven months earlier, it had taken me an extra hour to do the same.

'It's awful the way the time thing creeps in with running but you're only competitive against yourself. You like to see everyone doing well and competing. How they perform gives you an instant glimpse into how much they train.

'I have records of all my personal bests (PBs) on the computer. In 2002 I broke four hours with a time of three hours fifty-six and I still consider that one of my best achievements. My current PB is three hours twenty-six. I don't necessarily think you get faster over time but you get more interested and it's all down to training and experience, knowing what you're doing, getting the right surroundings, making sure you can get into the right frame of mind. It's exactly the same thing with business: understanding what you're doing and everything around you.

'The bottom line when you're running a business is that you have to look after yourself. If you make it a priority to look after yourself, there is more of a chance that you can help others around you. If you're unhealthy and smoking and overweight, you don't have the energy to do things. Running helped me to look after myself.

'I don't know where it's going for me with the running, to be perfectly honest. I've been increasing the number of marathons I've been doing each year, averaging between five and seven. This year I did ten in ten days at an event in England. That was the first big challenge. I went from a guy doing marathons to those who push it on another level. I was running marathons around Galway just to get in the miles. The training for that was really intense, horrific, but I would take weeks off in-between training sessions.

'When I'm not training, I feel really guilty, really down, but I get busy, dropping the kids around and that sort of thing. Since then I've signed up for the Marathon des Sables (a six-day endurance run across the Sahara Dessert covering a hundred and fifty-six miles). I saw the ten-day event as a stepping stone for training up to that.

'What I found in the early running stages was that I was no longer working late, I was out running. To get my training in I would have to be out at 5 pm and that meant people had to get along without me.'

THE CONNEMARA MARATHON
Sure enough Ray found time to discover and then develop the Connemara Marathon, which has since grown to be an international event, attracting more than three thousand runners annually.

'The Connemara Marathon just happened. I had decided to organise a marathon: I get these notions and this was the latest one. I discovered that organising a marathon is a huge amount of work. The first one – in 2001 – actually took place when I was on holidays. So a few people in Proactive got the word out for me.

'Altogether we had twelve people running the marathon and sixty running the half-marathon and something really special happened on that day. I had run five marathons at that stage but I didn't know a whole lot about the organisation involved or the detail you should look into. But I tried my best. Still, it was very strange for a guy like me on the starting line with eleven other people but all twelve of us gelled and we all seemed to know we were on the start of something really special. There was something in the air that morning that was just '"wow!"'

Indeed, the 'Connemarathon', as it has come to be known, became an overnight success. Enthusiasts in blogsphere all over the world rave about the wonderful scenery and magic attached to this event, which grows every year.

'I got in touch with Ireland West Tourism and wrote a proper business plan, calling it the Connemara International Marathon. From day one I had the sense it would become international. I estimated that we could have four hundred and fifty people running it by 2007 but six months later, when we held the second one, there were already six hundred and fifty in for it. So bang. It just exploded. We're expecting at least 3500 entrants for 2009.'

Ray believes that running a marathon is a fantastic achievement for anyone.

'It is special to run a marathon. If you tell anyone you ran a marathon, they'll sit up and listen. I've great respect for people who run 8k or 10k and then build up to a half-marathon if that's as far as they want to go. It's extraordinary that they can do that.

'What's happening now is that more and more people are doing marathons and there's a shift, so much so that the ultra-marathons (anything over 26.2 miles) now produce the "wow" factor. But ultra-marathons are hardly human! Can you imagine a bus going from Loughrea to Galway, dropping you off and telling you you have to run back again? That's what it's like!'

Did getting involved in the Connemarathon help Ray to become even more successful in his business?

'I think the Connemarathon has given me an awful lot. The first thing is, it's a hobby. It'll never be a money-making business because the logistics of getting all the people and the props out there are very costly. But it gives me a great buzz. When I come into work, I have design work to do and marketing plans. I'm the Creative Director so my work is about overseeing other designers and making sure everything is right. While all this is going on, I receive another entry for the Connemarathon and I'm constantly looking at where the participants are from. That happens twelve months of the year; last year we got entries for the 2009 event the day before 2008 entry closed. The half-marathon is where the mass market is because it's achievable by most people, as is a marathon. The difference is that people just don't have the confidence to do a marathon. Either way, at the finish line everyone gets a medal and a T-shirt and that's what it's all about.'

Ray regards the event as a lovely working partnership combining his hobby, his business life, team-building with colleagues and Proactive itself.

'The marathon has also been part of our team-building

here in the company as staff are all at the water stations on the big day and we have full production meetings here about how we're going to do things.

'Everyone has tasks. So it's a gel between my business life and my running. Among the staff now we have marathon runners and half-marathon runners. My brother Johnny completed a marathon in a second over three hours and our web designer has a 2.58 personal best. Others ran their first marathon never having achieved anything in running before and we also have one iron man (triathlon performer).'

Although Ray describes himself as someone who isn't very sociable, he agrees that he could talk about running for ever as it is his number one outlet in life.

'In my motivational speeches for Croi I enjoy telling people where my running started and where I'm going with it. My current goal is to run a hundred marathons by 2012. There's a club called the '100 Marathons' and once you do fifty marathons you can apply to be a 'wannabe' member. It's a worldwide UK-based organisation. I want to join that club. What will happen after that I don't know.'

Why does he want to do this?

'You have to have a goal or else you sink. Every challenge is just a stepping stone to the next challenge. I'm already looking at a few other milestones. I might go mad in 2010 and decide to do the remaining twenty or thirty marathons one after the other and get them out of the way. I'm looking at doing a hundred-mile race after that. I can't see any other sport to compare with running, although I do like swimming and I love climbing mountains too.

'It is scary territory because you do wonder when you are going to stop? Am I going to be a depressed fifty-five-year old who's done all he can do? It's great now because I have these goals and they're all achievable. That's how I look at it.'

How does Ray think running has helped him to develop as a person?

'Running has given me extreme calm and I can see that in the company as well. Before, I was aggressive. It was a case of "Don't touch Ray", "I'm too important." But now I'd like to think I'm much nicer. I'm not the tiger I used to be, always demanding control. It's a discipline you have to learn. You're going into work in the morning and you need to remember to bring your gear. You have to be organised. Before running, I definitely wouldn't have been organised.'

In addition to Proactive and Connemarathon, Ray is also the creator of a very successful on-line event-booking website entitled runireland.com, which organises entries for most high-profile races around the country.

'Maybe I had foresight when I discovered it was predominantly on-line entries that were coming through for the Connemarathon. I decided to drive all traffic online. Before that we had people ringing up asking a million questions and then there was the postal aspect to deal with. So we cut out all that administration and this year we're 100% online.

'I decided then to do the same for other races and set up runireland.com. I have one person here working on it full-time. It's not going to be a money-making business in itself but it generates other revenues, through races and events. It's also a way of expanding Connemarathon, which is really my baby. I can drive out there any time I like and once I'm on the route I feel at home.'

How did Ray happen upon the route for Connemarathon in the first place?

'That was an awful fluke. I grew up in Newcastle in County Galway and when we were kids, our parents often brought us to Oughterard. My mother, Noreena O'Connor, is an artist who paints mountains and landscapes and she always has a picture of the Connemara mountains in the house. One day I drove over to Peacocke's Hotel at Maam Cross, from where you can view the mountains, and I thought it would make a great finish for a marathon. Then I set the clock on the car to zero and by the time I had got to Leenane, it had clocked just over thirteen miles. I turned left and kept going until I made my way back to the hotel in a loop. The clock read twenty-six miles. That road was made for a marathon.'

Beautiful and scenic the Connemara Marathon may be but it is held in an isolated part of the country with few public amenities.

'The route has made life really difficult because there's no parking anywhere. This meant that we had to organise seventy-eight buses last year, which amounts to a lot of people to be moved around. The course has been the main problem.'

Still, it's all worth it as far as Ray is concerned.

'The Connemarathon gives me such a buzz because people are constantly entering and Proactive is still going strong. So it's a marriage of the two.'

Over the years Ray has kept a good note of his performance times, as much to keep himself motivated as to maintain a proper record.

'I achieved my personal best of 3.26 during the ten marathons in ten days event in May. The event is called the May Brathay Challenge and entails running ten times around the same marathon. It takes place on one of the toughest courses in Britain, in a place called Brathay in Cumbria. I decided to take my time on day one. I was really holding back and I kept that going for the first five days. I had had it in my head up to then that I could do three marathons in three days. I had already done two in two. My plan was to see if I could run five in five, then I would be on my way. So the sixth day was always going to be my wake-up call.

'In the end, I did them all in or around the same time, with a margin of about twenty minutes.

'The first five I did in 4.50, 4.46, 4.38, 4.20 and 4.20. I was running a little bit more freely there and managed 4.29 on the sixth day. There was a guy there trying to break the fastest record for the ten in ten who wanted to make 3.30 each day.

'It was a bit like Big Brother. There were eleven of us altogether, eight guys and three women. After the sixth day, the guy looking for the record was saying he was finding running on his own out front a bit lonely. So on the seventh day I decided I would go a little bit ahead and he could catch me up – but I didn't stop and that day I did a personal best of 3.26!

'I was on top of the world. The following day the same thing happened, I got home in 3.29. Then I picked up an injury on the ninth day: my ankle got busted up and I started to suffer. I did the race in 4.34 and took loads of painkillers on day ten, which was a full marathon with 1,000 people taking part.

'We got off an hour early and my ankle hurt so badly that I was munching painkillers. Going downhill was excruciating. As I passed the half-way point, the leader of the regular marathon went past me. The second guy tapped me on the back and the third the same. They were the elite runners and they were congratulating me, which gave me a lift. The next thing the pain disappeared. I did the second half in 1.50 and came home in 4.20. So 4.19 was my average.

'An awful lot of it was psychological. I couldn't get motivated to block the pain but as soon as I got a bit of a kick, it was gone. I enjoyed real euphoria after it but I was limping for three weeks. The pain was real and I was running the same pace as the elite women. I am a member of the Athenry Athletic Club where a lot of the elite runners are, so I never get cocky.'

You can get more information on the challenging, spectacularly beautiful Connemara Marathon on www. connemarathon.com

6

Ercus Stewart

Ercus Stewart is a senior counsel who has practised at the Bar since 1970. He is a keen cyclist, mountain runner and former Iron Man, having first discovered the world of fitness at the inaugural Dublin City Marathon in 1981. He celebrates his sixtieth birthday this year.

Ercus Stewart is a member of the Bars of England, Wales, Northern Ireland and New South Wales. He is also a Fellow of the Chartered Institute of Arbitrators, London, and an Arbitrator with the Court of Arbitration for Sport, which sits in Switzerland. He lectures in Arbitration Law and Employment Law in King's Inns and University College Dublin and was instrumental in the foundation of Just Sport Ireland, a national sports-dispute resolution body, as well as the Small Claims arbitration scheme. He has written three books and many articles and papers. Despite having such a heavy work schedule, Ercus has a personal best marathon time of three hours and four minutes and sill finds time to train by cycling most days from his home in County Wicklow to his work in the Four Courts in Dublin.

'I'm not mad into fitness but since my thirties I have been exercising fairly steadily. It started that day after I saw the first marathon being run in Dublin. I was sitting in a pub watching the six-hour people coming in, looking like death. I remember saying to myself, "I must do that next year."'

He began his training programme shortly afterwards.

'I started to train in Phoenix Park with my friend Noel. Our trick was to run three to four miles and then have three or four pints. Then I used to run with Donal, from up here beside me. He and I trained seriously so we did the second Dublin City Marathon in 1982 in a time of three hours twenty-one minutes.

'It was a lovely experience. Dublin is so hospitable, with so much good craic along the way. We finished at St Stephen's Green and as we walked into the park, I realised I couldn't lift my legs – I was so stiff after it all. But I was also exhilarated.'

The next day in the Four Courts Ercus could walk down the stairs only with great difficulty. 'That was new to me. The five or six months of training and the whole experience gave me a taste for fitness and I haven't stopped since.'

Between 1982 and 2006, Ercus ran a total of sixteen marathons throughout the world.

'Marathon running was at its height from the mid-1980s and I ran the London Marathon in 1985, 1986 and 1987, with a personal best time of three hours and four minutes. I also ran what was then the Limerick National Marathon and probably ran Dublin ten times altogether.

'In 1985 my friend Tom and I were on target to do New York in three hours and I'm sure we would have done it. But on the advice of a priest we met on the plane, who told us to drink pints and pints of orange juice, we both got sick – and I ended up finishing in three hours and nine minutes.

'The main reason it went wrong is because we spent the two

days before the event walking around enjoying a few drinks as we were made very welcome. That, combined with jet-lag and lack of sleep, did for us. But the New York Marathon really is a great one and the most sociable of all. I remember doing Paris the following year and it too was fantastic, just as I always found London to be. You wouldn't believe how enjoyable an experience it is.'

With a busy work schedule as an increasingly successful barrister, Ercus had to sandwich his training – which over time, graduated from distance running to mountain running and triathlon – between morning starts and evening closings.

'I had my first case at the Bar at twenty-one, which I suppose was young. I had thought about it in school and when I was fifteen I said I would be either a priest or a barrister. When people heard my barrister ambitions they said I was completely arrogant even to think like that. Nobody really went into the professions back then from where I was, an all-Irish Christian Brothers school. It was a very ordinary school and they didn't expect fellows like us to go to the Bar. It would have been seen as being above our station. But becoming a priest was acceptable.

'During my college years I wasn't really involved in sport or exercise at all but I enjoyed debating, student politics, languages, that kind of thing. I wasn't unfit either. I would have had a certain fitness because we had been walking five miles to school every day. People would give you a lift of course but in the country you were always active. So even though I didn't know it, I had kept a certain fitness. In college I know I put on some weight when I started drinking with the lads.

'For the first three years I didn't earn a penny at the Bar, which was normal. But it was very hard to keep going. I remember doing strange jobs to tide me over, including being a night watchman. I jacked it in to go off to Greece on a motoring trip with my brother.'

Ercus was thirty-two years old when he set his mind on running his first marathon.

'I took to running and regretted I hadn't done anything besides Gaelic football at school. In fact, they encouraged running in the school and there were running scholarships available back then to Villanova University in America. But they never encouraged me, whereas my brother Duncan did a bit of cross-country. I know now I was a better runner. I just wasn't aware of it then.

'I never cycled or swam as a child either. It all really changed that night in the pub. Up to then I had no interest in sport or fitness apart from what I watched on the box.'

Ercus started taking part in the Business Houses' League in Dublin, which usually consisted of five to six road races a year.

'Then the mountain running sucked me in and I still love it. I am often completely wrecked after a day's work in the city and feeling not fit to walk. But within ten seconds of the mountain race starting, the adrenaline is running and you instantly feel better.

'I discovered mountain running during my marathon training. I was running a mile and a half from my home and one of the local farmers said to me that there was a hill run being marked up on Kippure in the Wicklow mountains, where the RTÉ aerial is. I didn't know about mountain running or orienteering. I told my friend Donal and we went up and ran the whole thing the night before.

'We covered about eight to ten miles – distance wouldn't have been a problem for us by then, although for a non-hill-runner, the experience would probably be like being in a war-zone. We came back the next night and did the hill race and I was hooked. From then on, I ran the hill runs every Wednesday night of the May, June and July mountain-running calendar and except for when I was injured, I did them all most years since 1981.'

Even with mountain running in the bag, Ercus was still open to bigger challenges.

'A friend of mine, a lovely older man, asked me, 'Will you do a triathlon?' He had suffered a stroke but was still competing. I said I'd try. It entailed swimming half a mile in the sea, doing twenty-one miles on the bike and a ten-kilometre run. I had never swum any distance in my life – had never even done a length of a pool. All I ever did was plod around in water. I didn't even have a bike so I had to borrow one from my neighbours.

'There weren't any pedals on it and neither my friend Donal nor I were mechanical but somehow we got it going. It was a five-gear but I didn't dare change the gears once. I never even knew what gear I was on. After the cycle my legs were literally like jelly. I ran the ten-kilometre run with my legs feeling terrible. Then I was hooked on triathlons.'

Was the swimming part difficult?

'The first shock in the swim is you're with maybe a hundred people and they're all kicking and splashing in the open sea. Survive that! I'd recommend it to anyone, though, because it's really great.'

That first triathlon experience certainly didn't turn Ercus off: he was soon looking for similar events to compete in.

'There was a lot of triathlons being organised in the North of Ireland back then and that got me involved with people up there. In Craigavon and Belfast I did quite a few, eventually going for the All-Ireland Triathlon, which went from Greystones to Glendalough, with a sea-swim, fifty-six miles on the bike and a half-marathon run. I came twelfth in that but I'm not saying I was any good. There were only about thirty or forty people competing.

'Then I ran the All-Ireland in Sligo for the next ten years, covering the same distances. I did all ten of the All-Irelands and some other small triathlons, long and short, but Sligo was the most competitive. The winning time was usually around four hours and my time was around five hours. It was gruelling but I absolutely loved it. I was never a natural swimmer and was slow in the water but I used to make up the difference on the bike or running.'

By 1987 Ercus had graduated to the Iron Man event.

'This entailed swimming two-and-a-half miles in the sea, doing a hundred and twelve miles on the bike and running a full marathon. The event started at 6 am and you were required to wear wetsuits, which had been banned before – but the sea was just so cold.

'I came fourth in that but again it was no great achievement as there weren't that many in it. I wasn't doing it as a race and stopped and waited for the rest of our gang in the middle of it, drinking tea and eating sandwiches. Had I realised how far ahead I was and kept pressing on, I would possibly have come third.

'Again I remember that my legs were like jelly when I got off the bike after that event. A St John's Ambulance man told me to lie down on the road and this guy literally punished me by massaging my legs as hard as he could. As a result I was pain-free for the first fifteen miles of the run. But I do remember collapsing from hunger. I had to jog and walk it but I did that marathon in under four hours despite everything.

'So that was my path, from mountain running to triathlons and as a result, I became a cyclist, ultimately participating in some hundred-mile mara-cycles cross-border up to Belfast and back, through Sligo, Bundoran and Enniskillen. I did about four of those and they gave me another introduction to northern Irish people, Protestants and nationalists. There were no politics in it.

'Cycling remains my main interest today. I cycle in and out to work, which from the house is a twenty-six-mile round trip. I do it rain or snow and it's perfect for the times that are in it because it's energy-saving. I do it mainly because of the traffic because I can't stand sitting in a car in traffic. Apart from a puncture or the odd bit of danger from a few near misses, it's a joy. It means that as you come home after a day's work, you're already getting your exercise. Every workplace should have showers to help people become more active in this way. We now have showers in the Four Courts.'

A love of beautiful scenery adds to Ercus's enjoyment of his training runs and cycles. As he makes his way through the quiet back roads to one of the weekly runs between Glenasmole and Kippure organised by the Irish Mountain Running Association, he is an enthusiastic observer of the bog cotton.

'The whole bog is white. I love it. My mother once wrote a song about bog cotton that featured in the Castlebar Song Contest. The route here is over the Military Road, built to get at the rebels in west Wicklow after the 1798 Rising.

I've run the mountains of Ireland but never walked them. That's the funny thing, although I was reared in the Wicklow Mountains.

'Every Wednesday there's a run up one of the mountains here. I've been up here in peak snow, which isn't a very good idea on a racing bike. What drives me? Well, it's just mad. I know. But you want to get out. I don't like being indoors. I've no interest in sitting on machines in gyms and even swimming indoors doesn't appeal to me.

'It's the isolation I love. About twelve miles from my house, there isn't a house to be seen. I'm out here in rain, sleet or snow, usually on my own. That's not out of any mad wish to be on my own but it's just much easier organising yourself. Cycling and running you can do on your own and I wouldn't miss cycling by the old forest that belonged to the Guinness family, where you see no traffic on a week night, or doing a forty-mile round trip or going by Glendalough and Blessington, a trip of up to sixty-four miles.'

While he was pushing his body so hard, Ercus never considered whether his training was having any effect on his work performance.

'I would now look back and say, yes, it complemented my work performance because I don't think I could have kept doing all the hours or withstood all the pressure without the physical back-up that I have. I remember when I was in college a judge from England advising students to be fit, to have a healthy mind, a healthy body. It was even mentioned in our textbooks about how important it was to be fit at the bar.

'That wouldn't have made any impact on me then but clearly there are times when you are working terrible hours under huge pressure and fitness – getting fresh air into your system, getting your blood moving – is the key. It relaxes you, even if you don't switch off completely. I do believe fitness gets you through the tough times. I think it motivates you. A night like tonight, after that mountain run, you feel so much better. So in hard times it can help too. I'm hooked on it all, yes. I enjoy it. I started very badly. My breathing was bad. I had never been trained in running, in breathing, warming up or proper stretching. People who take up running need to know about these things and should make a conscious effort to work on them.

'I can remember ten years ago my brain was thinking arguments for a supreme court appeal as I cycled home. You don't want your brain to be working like this. I think I should forget things when I cycle – that's my whole plan. But I don't. Instead, my mind is clearing things out, uninterrupted.

'So I just took to hill running and cycling and still really enjoy it all. Even though I live beside the Wicklow mountains, it's not very convenient to get there when you're leaving the Four Courts and you are in the worst traffic you could imagine. That's why I started taking the bike to the hill-runs because it's easier to get there by bike than by car. In fact I'd be quicker getting out of the city than people in cars.

'I'm not doing anything like the running mileage now as my knees are causing a problem this year. So cycling is what I do most of all. My knee injury goes back to a skiing accident in 1991. I came off the mountain but nobody knew. I was in the middle of nowhere, somewhere in Austria. I lay there for half an hour.

'Eventually one of those tractors that go over the snow took me to hospital. Then I was sent home and operated on.

I was in hospital for a week and in plaster for eight weeks. When the plaster was taken off my leg was the worst thing I have ever seen. Just like a brush handle. There was absolutely no flesh: it was terrible to see it. I was like a famine victim.

'I had to do physiotherapy and, obviously, no running or cycling. Four months after the accident I tried the bike. Somebody had to hold it for me but I got back on and stayed there.'

Had he not discovered fitness, would he be the same man today?

'I'm not sure if there would have been any difference career-wise but from a social point of view, I suppose the time you spend running, you can't go drinking. I would have drunk a lot more if I wasn't running. I'm not at all anti-drink and I enjoy being social. I was part of the pub culture and am still perfectly happy to join the pub-drinkers but obviously I do it much less often. When I do it, I give it a good belt!

'I can recall on one occasion leaving a pub after two or three pints, going for a run, having a shower and returning to the pub. No one even noticed me gone but I had seven miles on them!'

On another occasion at a funeral in Booterstown, Ercus left the people he was with after three pints in order to run his weekly hill race.

'I ran it better because I was less fearful and suffered no after-effects. But I'm not advocating drinking and running of course.'

Shortly after he took up his training, Ercus made major progress in his career.

'I was a barrister in 1970 and became a senior counsel in 1982, which was around a year after I started my running. I'm at it since so I've now been thirty-eight years in the law.'

Has the legal profession changed much over the years?

'Well, I'm probably too long at the job now to think about doing something else but yes, definitely, it has changed. It is much more dog-eat-dog. There's not nearly the same camaraderie or spirit there and it's not the same good life as it used to be, in the sense that we don't even go for a cup of coffee and some craic with the pals. It's not happening now because everyone is too busy.

'It's also much more cut-throat as regards clients and cases. Obviously now there's a lot more barristers. When I started there were about two hundred barristers in the country but now there's an awful lot of young barristers without any business at all. So there would be a lot of poverty in the Bar today.'

During his early career in law, Ercus discovered an interest in socialism and was soon representing the underprivileged in Irish society.

'While I was in college I got involved in debating and then went into left-wing politics. In 1968 I went to America and started to think. I spent a short period in Harlem and saw conditions that were a lesson to me. I worked outdoors in Rhode Island for my first year, during the year of the presidential election campaign against Nixon. I took quite an interest and was greatly influenced by an Irish-American professor in the house. I started reading up on things.

'I came back to college and joined the Labour Party. It didn't help me in my career and if anything, it would have been a huge hindrance in the early years. But through the Party, I began to take an interest in social work and charity work. It wasn't so much charity as doing things. About ten of us had a little group called 'Action' and we used to go to the slums in Dublin and cook and clean flats for old people. I remember the conditions there, young girls unable to get the fleas out of their hair. It was absolute filth.

'The other thing we went into was teaching kids English, Irish and Arithmetic, down in Sherriff Street, in the north inner city, near where the IFSC is located – it was a real slum then. We used to get a room in Liberty Hall. The kids always called us "Brother". We taught them those subjects on week nights.

'When I finished my Bar finals I worked in America for more than four months and planned to go on to Mexico to work in an orphanage. But that didn't work out because of my visa. I returned home to do the call to the Bar. You can't practise unless you're called. When I came home I got a telephone call that some of the kids we had been teaching in Sherriff Street had been arrested.

'I didn't even know there was such a thing as children's courts. I was completely ignorant. These six kids were up for having tried to burn their school. I was asked to defend them. There was no legal aid so these kids from all over Ireland just came before these courts. Clearly there was no defence for them so they would end up being found guilty and locked up in places like Letterfrack Industrial School in County Galway. They could be sent there for two or three years – even up to seven years. I've seen innocent children locked up in these places for as long as nine years.

'I said, "Well, I can't defend them. I haven't been called to the Bar." I was very nervous about what I could do because I was very ignorant. We adjourned the case for two weeks and got an instructing solicitor. I came back and represented them and with hinting and help from the solicitor, who was more experienced than me, I got the six kids got off.

'Because of this, more and more kids started asking me to defend them and I took on their cases. I didn't realise it was helping me in that I was learning and learning. I believed every kid, even though they couldn't all have been telling the truth. But I believed them, which meant I thought the guards were all wrong. That meant I cross-examined the guards and it would be pretty hard cross-examination as they were clever guards and I was relatively inexperienced.

'So I spent a year supposedly devilling but I wasn't really devilling, I was defending kids in the children's court and I suffered nightmares because I was frightened and inexperienced. But as a result I became very good at criminal law, criminal defence and cross-examination. I loved it at that stage. I was driven; I was idealistic.

'I then started taking test cases for children, or on behalf of adults, on things such as the right to free legal aid, the right to be informed of free legal aid, and on the charge of vagrancy or loitering with intent. I challenged that law and maybe five or six others. We lost the cases in the High Court but won them in the Supreme Court. That brought an end to those laws, yes.

'Then we won entitlement to criminal legal aid for everybody. Obviously the problem now is that it is given too easily to ruthless criminals rather than genuine cases but you will always find that reform benefits the bad as well as the good.

'Then I did some cases on illegitimacy and the right of the illegitimate child to succeed. We lost in the High Court and the Supreme Court. I brought in Mary Robinson, because she was senior to me, and we went to Strasbourg on that and won. So I did all that kind of stuff in the 1970s. I was more motivated and idealistic back then and became very interested in Constitutional Law.'

During his years as a junior counsel Ercus practised criminal law and then family law, before taking silk (becoming a senior counsel) in 1982.

'I did all these awful cases for which there was no income, no legal aid – a lot of them went free, 'pro bono' or whatever. And I did some ordinary civil claims. At that time I was one of the top three criminal barristers, I would have been the top barrister in family law.

'I took one family case for an old client after I took silk. She had lost her children because she was in an adulterous relationship. The law in Ireland was against the woman because she was in a relationship with another man and this was very much frowned upon. I handled that on appeal in the Supreme Court and she won.

'That was the only family case I took since I took silk, even though I devoted a huge amount of my time to it before that. With regard to criminal cases, I took one murder case that year as well – 1982. The defendant was found guilty of manslaughter, not murder.'

Does he defend people he knows are guilty?

'If you're a barrister, you know what's happening. If they say, "I'm guilty, I did such and such," you can't put them in the witness box to tell a lie. But you can still defend them to the best of your ability. And you do. It's easier to defend a fellow you know to be guilty because you don't have any interest in him, whereas if I believe you're innocent and I defend you, I'm not as good a performer because I'm not objective, I'm subjective. I'm interested in the case and trying to win it.

Clinically you do better as a criminal lawyer if you actually hate your client. It's true.

'Criminal law is just a job. It's the easiest job because there's no night work in it, there's no paper work in it, no research. Of course there are ethics. The ethics are that you don't put your client in the witness box to say something that he has told you the opposite of. But it's up to the state to prove the case. It's not up to you to convict. Even if I believe you are guilty, you're still entitled to a defence. In the end I gave up criminal cases because I was probably getting too many people off who were guilty.'

Having given up criminal law, Ercus concentrated on family cases and also did a lot of civil and employment cases.

'And now I do arbitration, including my work at the Court of Arbitration for Sport in Switzerland which tackles sporting disputes. My own involvement in sport and arbitration gave me the interest. It would include challenges to race records, drug abuse charges, that kind of thing. Recently I did a case in Ireland about an Olympics sporting dispute. After a week of 6 am starts through to 10.30 pm, we won that case. I do commercial arbitration as well as sports arbitration. I also got involved in teaching lawyers in Africa as they didn't have the skills to defend clients.'

Ercus celebrates his sixtieth birthday this year, but shows no signs of slowing down.

'Yes, I'm going into a new category this year, the sixty- to seventy-year-olds, so I'll probably become competitive again. I'm quite interested in that. Unfortunately, I've two very bad knees at the moment so I'm back with the walking wounded.

'I'm in the Irish Triathlon Association and the Irish

Mountain Running Association but you don't train or run with these associations. I'm not in a club as such. My training has changed over the years, of course. Obviously, for the marathons, I was doing huge mileage. I'd be running nights, weekends and putting in a few extra hours in the week to put up the mileage. I continued with that for more than fifteen years.

'Now I do almost no running training. I do my hill running once a week in the summer and usually improve on that each week but my cycling is what's building me up. If I was to take it really seriously I would have to do more training but I just don't have the time. It's a fifty-minute cycle into work and if I come home again on the bike it's an hour-and-a-half, because it's uphill, so even doing that each day takes a lot of time.

'But when I can get away at all, I do. All I ever have with me is a bottle of water. I've never taken gels. I had to go to an arbitration in Vienna and after that took my bike on the train to the ski resort where my family was staying for the week. When they went home I cycled from the resort down to Salzburg, staying a night in a guest house above a pub, before finally making my way to Budapest.

'After a vicious night of drinking until 4 am, a horrible breakfast I couldn't eat, washed down by two cups of coffee, one bun and a big bottle of soft drink, I finally reached Budapest. I had done a hundred and forty miles on the bike with nothing to eat. I thought it was only a hundred miles. It was just too early to go back!

'You never worry when you're cycling or running. You're just happy to do it. These activities have changed my life and I don't see myself stopping them. Definitely exercise has kept me young. I didn't believe I was competitive. I never did hill runs competitively. Once I won a hill run by default because visibility was so bad that the fellows ahead of us got lost and I sprinted ahead of my friend at the end and came first! That happens in hill running.

'Coming down a mountain on the bike is worse because cow dung or anything can make the road very slippery. I've skidded down a few times and the mountain was vicious. If a car comes by you're really in trouble. I was coming across once to train and was tied on to the bike with toe clips. Just as a car passed my rucksack fell off and I keeled over trying to get it. The driver must have thought I was a basket case.

'I didn't realise I was competitive until I turned fifty and I was running up Carrantouhill. A guy from Limerick kept asking me what age I was. I didn't realise he was fifty and that he wanted to win the category. In the end I came second, because a dark horse turned up from England and he was a very good runner and won the category. So I was second to him. I don't realise it until I start but I am very competitive.'

Still, it must be nice to win a medal or two.

'When I realised that I was featuring in races, from then on I did take a bit of an interest and I've started watching other guys the same age as me. I won the Irish Mountain Running Championship in 1999 and three other years. That doesn't mean much because the good guys don't run them all but I still won the championship and the league and that is quite a nice thing to do.

'Basically, you'd know people of your own age-group, you'd watch them, they'd watch you. So it was very competitive amongst our age-group. The only trouble is, as you head towards your sixties, there are much younger runners in your category and the standard now is much higher than when I fifty. The runners of fifty and fifty-one are much better runners. I'm giving that away against myself that I was winning when the competition wasn't as severe. The really top guys, they're incredible, they're like deer. It's an Olympic sport and they take it very seriously.

'It's the same thing with cyclists, by the way. I don't do any racing with my cycling, only as part of the triathlons. But there's a Veteran Cyclists' Association. I'm a member but not a participant. The old guys can do it because they're experienced as hell.'

7

Catherine Wiley

Catherine Wiley (née Denning), is a native of Castlebar, County Mayo. She married her husband Stewart when they were both in their twenties and together they built up one of the most successful travel businesses and children's camp operations in Europe, Camp Beaumont. Catherine has been a constant charity worker over the years, fund-raising and campaigning on behalf of Romanian orphans and the underprivileged. Most recently, she has taken on the cause of grandparents, who she believes are under-appreciated in modern society. She was instrumental in setting up the first ever Grandparents' Day in Ireland in 2007, and this is now an annual event.

Catherine's interest in keep-fit was sparked when she hit her late forties and noticed the first signs of physical decline, including severe osteoporosis. It was at this time also that, with regard to her business and other comitments, she drew breath for the first time in years. Since then she has incorporated regular workouts into her life and plans to continue holding on to her two original knees, despite medical advice to the contrary.

Her approach is very holistic, in that she uses her fitness

workouts as part of her work-life balance for body, mind and spirit. Crucially, Catherine sees fitness as a hugely effective tool against the stresses of life, when things are really getting you down.

'When people are struggling, if only they knew how helpful it is to exercise.'

Catherine's calling is clearly towards altruism. While she did spend years building up a successful business, success and money have never been her true motivation. Instead, she has been driven all her life to help people who need help.

It is evident that, while fitness is important to Catherine as she gets older, it is more a tool she uses in order to follow her passions in life. Her work clearly comes second, as one telling comment from Catherine reveals.

'At a very early age I decided that I would be useful wherever I went in the world.'

The reason Catherine discovered the world of fitness relatively late in life was that she had always been so busy and active with her work.

'I never needed fitness in my early life because I was always very energetic. I had a very busy office life and social life and it never occurred to me to do anything recreational to keep myself physically fit, because I was running up and down the stairs and looking after the kids. Also, I was very fortunate that I never had a weight problem – it was never difficult for me to be slim. But fitness became an important contributor to my mental ability as I grew older.

'You know, I think people experience changes of life without even realising that they have started happening to them. For me, it all began with the *Challenge Anneka* project on TV, a campaign headed up by the TV personality Anneka

Rice to restore an orphanage in Romania and give the kids a Christmas party. I took part in that project and I have been active in it ever since, going on for eighteen years at this stage.

'When I started doing that, my husband and I were already running a very successful business. I had left Ireland at the age of fourteen, with no education except the little I got from the Sacred Heart school in Westport.

'I went working in England, lying about my age, as you do, to get jobs. Then when I was twenty-one I met Stewart and we started a company, Corfu Villas, which was a precursor to the opening up of the Greek islands as holiday destinations. All the villas we operated were leased – we owned nothing – and from that, we started a huge operation.

'We met a lot of people along the way and gradually our Corfu base extended until the company grew to become Greek Island Holidays, and from there, we graduated to Camp Beaumont. Summer camps were a way of life in the US and basically, with Camp Beaumont, we brought the concept to the UK.'

Catherine initially became aware of the summer camp phenomenon from her own family experiences.

'I had two children of my own and then two stepchildren with Stewart, who had been married before. I was amazed when I learned that my two stepchildren were going to summer camp in America, because I had never heard of the concept. The camp they went to was the YMCA and my own children started going there too.

'You could go for one week, two, three or whatever and each week would have a different theme, depending on where the camp was. So you could have arts and crafts one week, then archery, judo and all sorts of sporting activities.

'I had always been a working mother and I know the needs and demands that go with that. You have to figure out how to keep the children occupied and at the same time not just dump them somewhere that leaves them feeling they are being dumped. You have to be very careful.

'We brought the concept of American-style summer camp to Britain more than thirty years ago – it also spread to Ireland. We started Kids Summer Camps, day and residential. We went on to develop International Language Schools, then year-round residential educational centres. We started the first computer camps. All these were linked to the UK's national curriculum. We became one of the biggest providers of school education journeys in the UK. When we sold the company three years ago we were dealing with nearly four hundred thousand children a year.

'The reason we called it Camp Beaumont was because the first camp was based in Beaumont. We lived in London in those days and Camp Beaumont grew and grew. In reality we started an entirely new industry. Within ten years, I suppose, we had about fifteen camps and were taking about 30,000 children a year.

'We went from Camp Beaumont day camps to residential camps, where children came and stayed for a week or two weeks. A lot of parents did this as a prelude to boarding school, bringing their children to the camp to try out the experience. Some of them were quite young, only six or seven.

'In the early days, I worked at the camps on a round-the-clock, twenty-four-hours-a-day basis. I was all over the place like a lunatic. Obviously there was no need for me to work at keeping fit then but I was promoting fitness at every level, because all our camps had two components, education and physical exercise. So there was a balance.

'During the day the children would learn about computers or science or the environment for a couple of hours, then they would spend the rest of the time doing sports and activities.

'After that we set up English-language schools and I travelled extensively, setting up agencies all over the world. We brought children over to the UK from everywhere.

'Then we went into Kingswood, which was purely educational. This happened after we started to buy up our own schools. Boarding schools were not flavour of the month back then as people were having second thoughts about sending their children to them because of scandals and reports of paedophiles. So we bought quite a number of boarding schools. I think we ended up with fifteen of them. We started them off again with our own brand of new programmes. European and overseas kids from as far away as Argentina would come for three to four weeks and learn a language and integrate with other kids for cultural reasons.

'We also expanded into the year-round school market, offering school trip visits, so teachers from all over the UK came with classes of kids on an ongoing basis. We still have more than a dozen London day-camps in operation today, thirty years later.'

Catherine has always had the mind of a businesswoman and continues to spot new opportunities.

'If I walk down the street I'm getting ideas, I'm dangerous that way. The fact is, ideas are all around you. You don't have to reinvent the wheel. It's already there. You just have to avail of it.'

Not only did Camp Beaumont provide Catherine with

the perfect opportunity to develop a multi-million-pound business from scratch, the nature of the business encouraged her altruistic side.

'Running Camp Beaumont, it gave me a tremendous vehicle to do things with my life that I would never had the opportunity to do. For example, when I started going to Romania, more than twenty years ago, it was during Nicolae Ceauşescu's regime, which was very corrupt, so it was very hard to get anything done.

'But because I had Camp Beaumont, I could bribe officials by offering their kids English-language stays at Camp Beaumont or, if the kids were older, offering them a job.

'It opened so many doors in that way and over the years we brought hundreds of kids from Romania. Nobody needed to know about this because it was a private initiative. It was no big deal. It was just that the company enabled me to do it.

'Wherever I went in the world, I wanted to be useful. If I was in Japan or Cambodia, for example, I would always find a priest or an orphanage that I could help. I honestly don't know why I was like this. Maybe it has to do with how we are brought up.

'I've always been extremely comfortable with all kinds of people, poor or rich, famous or not. As a result of my experiences in Romania, I decided to go back to college and ended up doing two degrees in psychology. I was facilitating lots of adoptions and people started coming to me for advice on child development, cognitive behaviour and all that and I felt I needed to understand child development.

I believe everybody has their own drive. It's how you put that drive to use that matters, the same as with anything else.

For me, there have always been two loves in my life: one is kids, the other is old people.'

As well as being driven with regard to her business and charitable work, Catherine has always maintained a disciplined approach to her life.

'That's where I think exercise comes in for me. It is all about discipline. When people go to the gym and see a good figure, they wonder: how did she get that? Well, they can do it too if they just have the right attitude, the ability to discipline themselves.

'People use all kinds of excuses not to exercise but the truth is that we all have struggles in our lives and I would suggest that if we do have problems, the ability to exercise and focus on that exercise helps us enormously. Of course there are excellent resources such as Alcoholics Anonymous for alcohol abuse or Gamblers Anonymous for gambling addicts. But the answer is always within yourself.

'The reality is that we're very caught up with ourselves these days. Everyone seems to think it's all about them. Society encourages people to be like this. If I thought like that all the time I couldn't cope. People are putting themselves before commitment but the reality is that you have to make commitments first, even if it is only a commitment to behave in a particular way for a month.

'Through my company we helped people in Vietnam, India, Cambodia – wherever I happened to be. Eventually I developed my own charity, for want of a better word. I became a grandparent and started looking at the needs of grandparents, after recognising what a huge transition it is to become a grandparent.

'Grandparenthood just happens to you. One minute you're

raising your children and it's all about time, recipes, nutrition. They are your focus. But this changes completely when you become a grandparent.

'For some people being a grandparent is fabulous but for others it is very challenging. What with marital breakdown, drug addiction, single-parent families and people living to be much older than in previous generations, grandparents have to face problems they would never have thought of.

'They end up picking up the slack and whatever extra money they have, they are expected to spend it on their grandchildren's education, clothes and birthdays. I know many grandparents would be terrified to say this, so I'll say it on their behalf.

'It's also a real dilemma for grandparents today: knowing when to give advice, when to step away, where to draw the line. They are afraid they'll hurt someone's feelings. There are often many people in the family equation, including two sets of grandparents, one being played off against the other.

'While I started Grandparents' Day for schools in 2008, my Grandparents' Pilgrimage started in England six years ago. The basic idea was very simply to honour St Joachim and St Anne, Mary's parents and the grandparents of Jesus. I felt there was no better way of bringing faith up to date in relation to grandparents.

'We started a pilgrimage to honour and give thanks to grandparents for all they've done down through the ages for us. Our pilgrimage continues to this day because grandparents are so undervalued, even though they really are faith in action. They genuinely don't realise all the good they are doing because being a grandparent is so rooted in love. Often they have a much better relationship with their grandchildren than they had with their own kids; that's because they have more time to enjoy them. They are also more tolerant and much wiser. It's really much easier to be a grandparent than a parent and they can also be a great source of joy to the parents – their own children – who know they can rely on them for their kids, even if that may not have been the case when they themselves were growing up.'

Catherine initially tried out the Grandparents' Day idea in England but found it was 'like pulling teeth'.

'Even though it has cost me a fortune in the UK and sometimes fewer than a hundred people attend, the event is still growing and everybody who does turn up for the day loves it and begs me not to give it up. But then I hit on the notion that it would probably go down fantastically well in Ireland. It all started in Knock, after Archbishop Michael Neary held a diocesan meeting to involve lay people more in the Church, because of lack of vocations. I managed to get myself invited along because of my dreams for the Grandparents' Day but of course, grandparents weren't on the agenda. I was wondering: what am I doing here?

'I decided that I would not leave until I had told somebody about the Grandparent Pilgrimage idea. I left the meeting but wrote to the Archbishop, promising him that if he would lead the pilgrimage, I would give all my time over the coming year to it. The archbishop replied that he would be delighted to lead it and that was the start of it.

'On the first official Grandparents' Day in 2007, 5000 people attended and we launched our Children's Prayer, asking all grandparents to write a prayer for their grandchildren. I also wrote to the Pope asking him to offer his blessing to the pilgrimage and to write a prayer, because I couldn't find one that supported, encouraged and acknowledged grandparents and their great value, worth and effort. When you think about it, even godparents get some glory at baptisms but where do grandparents get the glory? Where do they fit in their own right in the family? It's not like it used to be in the olden days, with Granny and Grandad sitting by the fire and us looking after them. People seem to have very little time to spend with their families now.

'I felt there really was a need for the role of grandparents to be reaffirmed. I contacted Rome, heard nothing and then went and visited myself. I brought a whole sheaf of prayers written by children in Ireland. At the Vatican they told me that it was likely the Pope would never write a poem for grandparents. I insisted. I believed that if he could just see the children's prayers, he too would write a prayer. Two minutes later the Holy Father wrote the prayer and it's the best prayer ever, one that honours grandparents.'

Catherine acknowledges that her faith is more important than ever in her life as she grows older.

'I definitely find it grows as you get older. When I was younger I used to think my own mother was a religious fruitcake, because her faith was so strong. Now it's a case of my chickens coming home to roost, because so many people I've been meeting are priests!'

Catherine's own fitness routine is fairly disciplined, constituting daily workouts either in the gym or at fitness classes.

'I live in Lecanvey outside Westport when I'm home in Ireland and my personal trainer (Paul O'Brien, who also features in this book) comes out at 8.30 am. We have a small gym in the house. I go through my paces with Paul for forty-five minutes, then I have a shower and go to Mass.

'I consider that I'm holistically well looked after, body and soul then, so normally I'll go to the office after that. I travel extensively all the time, so this fitness routine is very important to me. I think the reason people fall off the wagon with business is lack of routine. You have to have routine in your life, just as when you were a child. If you deviate from the script, you head towards imbalance. Of course you'll wrong-foot yourself from time to time, such as when you sit on the wrong side of a car in a new country, but it's about finding a rhythm that suits you. If you really want to become serious, you have to get in with the rhythm of life.'

At her second home in America, Catherine takes a different approach to her fitness routine, relying on set classes to keep her going.

'I have to go to classes because I need motivation. Although I'm a highly motivated person, I still need the input of other people to get me going. America has an awful lot to offer in terms of physical health education for older people and I'm definitely at the younger end of my class's age-group.

'I go every morning to a class called twenty/twenty, which includes aerobics, weights and core and abs exercises. For me the classes are very important. Quite seriously, I don't think I could survive without them or without going to the gym. I'm lucky to be able to have a trainer and I would make other sacrifices in order to be able to afford one.'

Catherine believes that what we must fight against at all times is stress. Fortunately, there are many ways we can do this.

'You can help yourself so much just by doing exercise. The chemicals in your body actually change when you exercise. The endorphin hormone is released in your brain. Just imagine all the blood in your circulation being clogged and furred up. Then think about how exercise will get everything moving properly again. Wouldn't you be mad not to do it.

'Exercise is an essential ingredient for good health and for life. The stresses in your life may feel like as if they are just mental but anyone with an ounce of sense knows that psychological stresses have physiological outcomes. If you're harbouring something in your mind, it has to manifest itself in some way in your body.'

Conscious that she is getting older, Catherine intends to live as long as possible and wants to hold on to as much of her original body as possible for as long as she can!

'I went to a doctor a couple of years ago and he said I needed two new knees. I'm not ready for them yet so I thought: what can I do? I know, I'll strengthen my calf and thigh muscles. I thought that if I did this, I could leave it longer before having my knees done. By the time I have to get them done, medicine will be so much better and the new knees they give people will last much longer.

'In fact, after the pilgrimage in Knock, I really suffered with my knees. I knew I pushed myself beyond my limits, just working on the project, and bit by bit, my body deteriorated. I had to get injections in my knees and then my back went. I'd been carrying a lot of stress with it all – as I say, stress will catch up with you if you don't manage your life properly.'

As an 'oldie' of sorts herself, Catherine acknowledges that older people can be extremely competitive and won't hold back just because their bodies have been through the mill.

'I think peer pressure is just as important for older people as it is for young people. If you really want to make your body look a certain way, you can. You just need to project that image of yourself a month forward, telling yourself you'll look the way you want to then. You imagine yourself having stuck to the fitness regime and the diet. This is all good for you and it helps you to reach your goal. But nothing works better than being told you need two new knees!'

Unfortunately, it isn't only her knees that trouble her: Catherine's entire skeletal system is off kilter.

'I have the worst form of osteoporosis you could ask for but the way I see it, I'm strengthening my skeletal system by adhering to my fitness routine. People can either sit back and moan or get on with it. It's all about having a positive attitude. You can only deal with what comes to you but if you have the right attitude of mind, you'll be fine. Attitude is nature combined with nurture. It's certainly learned. But the best thing I learned in psychology is that while everything is leaned, it can also be unlearned.

'My friend was attending bereavement counselling and I said to her to try and get some exercise. Exercising does a great deal for older people. What we need is peer-group activity – people who go into old people's homes and start exercise classes. You need people on TV talking about exercise as well as visible role models at all times.

'People talk about needing expensive equipment or not wanting to go to the gym but actually, you don't have to have anything to get fit. The gym I go to here will show you a twenty-minute mobile routine that suits people who travel. You can do your squats while brushing your teeth.'

Since developing osteoporosis, Catherine has also learned of the many benefits of resistance training.

'I never realised how important resistance training was

until the last few years. Once you get beyond concentrating on weight loss, after you get fit, what people really envy is your disposition. The truth is that people should never focus on weight loss. Weight's got nothing to do with it. What we should be concentrating on is how to get people in old people's homes fit and at what age they should still be strengthening their bones with weight training. The great thing about weight training is that the muscles take a long time to forget. They have a very good memory so you can always come back to the exercises if you miss a few weeks.

'If I go two to three weeks without doing any exercise, that would be my absolute limit. I won't let it go past that and for the rest of my life, I do not see it stopping. There are all sorts of precautions you can take if you are physically handicapped in some way. I do realise there are certain things people are not able to do but even in a wheelchair, you can exercise. When it comes to fitness, you can always do something.'

With official pension age now creeping up on her, Catherine has no intention of slowing down.

'I've never worked harder in my life. I love my life although I do get anxious sometimes and think perhaps I've bitten off more than I can chew. If I was working for money I'd be a multimillionaire ten times over. Happily, my husband totally supports what I am doing now with my life and because I am not in it for the money, I don't take anything remotely personally.

'I am so thrilled that 10,000 people turned up at Knock for this year's Grandparents' Pilgrimage Day. It was only our second year and I feel we're just starting to get the message out.'

Catherine has now set her sights on getting grandparents

around Ireland to walk the length and breadth of the country in the name of charity!

'I'm looking now to do a sponsored walk for grandparents. The aim would be to try and get houses for the millions of African grandparents who are bringing up their own grandchildren because the children's parents have died of AIDS. To do the event, Irish grandparents would have to get into training, They would have to get fit! Let's see where that takes us. If it's a runner, maybe it could become an annual event!'

And if this doesn't work out, Catherine has another novel idea to set up 'granny camps', that would operate along the same lines as the children's camps!

'I hope the Grandparents' Pilgrimage will be a worldwide mission, encouraging grandparents everywhere to transmit the faith.'

Any other plans after that?

'Oh, yes. I just think, please God that it will continue indefinitely until I drop. Then just lay me out in Chanel and say, "You've done a great job" – and I'll be happy!'

Further information on grandparents' day is available on www.nationalgrandparents.com

8

David Hegarty

As we have seen from the interviews in this book, fitness fanatics who love their hard-core workouts and sweaty sessions in the gym often attribute their success in life and productivity at work to the fact that they keep their bodies in peak physical condition. Physical fitness clearly provides people with a powerful life-management tool; consequently, during these current recessionary times, getting fit could be a worthwhile investment for many.

Indeed, those in the business of counselling and life-coaching are now strongly recommending fitness as a way forward for people. The message is basically that while the world around us may be spinning out of control, at least we still retain the power to control our physical selves.

In response to this state of affairs, we should ensure that our bodies are strong, fit and in the best condition that they can be, as a defence against any hard knocks that may be coming our way. No matter how bad our personal situation may become, by being fit and primed for action, we will be able to face up to life's challenges and have the energy to address them proactively.

YOGAMETRICS

There are many roads to peak physical fitness. While most fitness fanatics tend to follow the route of hard-core aerobic and resistance-training workouts, there are alternative, gentler approaches that also promise physical fitness as a reward.

Yoga is one such discipline, which centres around drawing people's attention to the functioning of their bodies in relation to posture, breathing and movement. Some people have the mistaken idea that yoga is based on complicated movements and positions and suitable only for the very flexible among us. Happily, there are many practitioners in the world of yoga who want to make it accessible to everybody. Indeed, just concentrating on breathing and posture goes a long way towards helping people to develop physical fitness, as one leading fitness guru in Dublin has demonstrated to thousands of clients over the years.

This individual is David Hegarty, who devised a fitness system of his own based on yoga over thirty years ago, which he named 'yogametrics'. This system, claims David, can help people cope with every kind of stress life throws at them, even an economic crisis such as the global recession affecting the population at large today.

What is particularly interesting about David's yogametrics and the 'dynamic health system' he developed subsequently is their simplicity. They don't entail long, hard workouts that leave the body lathered in sweat. Instead, they require the practitioner to adopt good posture and engage in regular, gentle breathing exercises while making a commitment to being constantly aware of how the body is feeling and reacting as it carries out its normal activities.

The *lack* of vigorous exertion entailed in this system may

seem ridiculous to those who swear by hard-core workouts for fitness, but, having practised some of the basic breathing exercises myself, I can already see why it might work. David explains that the basis of its success is that full and proper breathing helps to circulate rich, oxygenated blood right around the body, making everything work more efficiently. He adds that the reason that exercise and fitness workouts make people feel good is that it is often only during their workouts that people really breathe deeply and correctly.

It is important to note that the 'body awareness' commitment made by practitioners of David's system should ideally be applied to every movement of the body from dawn to dusk, to ensure that all body movements are thought through and performed with the utmost efficiency. This awareness generates an optimum performance level in the body, in relation to the basics of breathing, posture and the ongoing circulation of rich oxygenated blood.

Of course, it isn't possible for any of us to be 100% aware of all our thoughts and actions twenty-four hours a day, or even during our waking hours. So busy is our world today that for many of us each day passes in a blur. It's asking a lot of us to take time out to become deliberately conscious of how we are feeling and what we are doing.

Bearing this in mind, David devised a system that requires a minimum time commitment of ten to fifteen minutes a day of practitioners. It may seem like a paltry amount of time to dedicate to self-improvement. In reality, however, a ten-minute window in your day devoted to making yourself feel better, in which you can focus entirely on yourself without interruption, may well be very hard to find. If you take the trouble to fit this 'me time' into your day, it can have a tremendously beneficial effect on your wellbeing in the long run.

This has been the finding of the many clients over the years who have adopted David's yogametrics and dynamic health system – which also advocates a nutritious diet and the avoidance of stress – and who swear by it as a life-management and fitness regime.

Describing each person as 'their own greatest asset', David maintains that it is important to concentrate on learning how to be well in order to be well. His system, he claims, helps people to lose excess weight, manage stress, invigorate the system, tone the abdominal wall, firm up slack muscle and flatten the stomach. David says:

'Being fit and well is a skill, like playing an instrument. As with learning to swim or ride a bike, it can be learned and then practised, simply. Once people do this, they can get on with their lives, better equipped to cope and live.'

David adds that fitness is key to good health: 'We have more influence over our health than we realise. Some people exist, others live. The difference is often a simple matter of fitness. The choice is nearly always yours.'

Noting that not everyone has the time or the inclination to sit in traffic on the way to a gym, queue for their turn on equipment, battle their way through congested swimming pools, or run around the streets at six in the morning, David espouses yogametrics as the perfect solution.

'Yogametrics can be practised in the car, the kitchen, the office, the workshop, the hotel room or the gym. You take it with you wherever you go. It is used by people from the age of fifteen to eighty-plus. It is the skill of using the natural resources that are available to everyone, all the time. It effectively turns every activity into a beneficial exercise.'

Everyone has the right to be as well as they can, David believes.

'As an individual, you are your own greatest asset. I believe that asset should be given every chance to flourish.

'Yogametrics teaches how to turn the body into a trim, fit, naturally well, health-promoting unit. You don't have to be a fanatic. If you want the energy, the wellness, the sense of vitality that comes from being basically fit, and if you harness that desire to learn and practise some basic principles, it's almost physically impossible not to get a good result. Yogametrics will help you to create a fitness for life, establish a normal body weight and a real sense of wellbeing. I believe everyone owes themselves that chance.'

Strong talk. Irrespective of whether David's health systems appeal to the fitness fanatic in you, or whether he convinces you it's worth giving them a shot, David Hegarty certainly has a lot of expertise to offer in regard to physical health after forty years in the business. You can read more about his fitness systems in his book *Dynamic Health*.

David, why is your health system entitled 'yogametrics'?

'It's a little play on the word yoga, as it combines elements of yoga with some simple physical exercises. For years I myself practised yoga and I still adhere to the principles of it.

'But there was always something about yoga that was shrouded in mystery. It was a little bit elitist, I thought, and I felt the practitioners were interested in you only if you were into very advanced methods. They'd say to me: you don't know what you're talking about. But I got a lot of positive vibes from just practising the simple stuff myself, certain poses that tap into what's known as the prana, or life-force energy.

'So I just changed the language and did a play on words, to make yoga accessible to everybody as part of a method of getting fit.

'The fact is that a lot of people train very well and religiously, perhaps three to four times a week, but many of them overlook the fact that their posture and breathing aren't right while they're working out. As a result of this they may be missing a huge proportion of the benefits they should be enjoying.

'Also, people often go from one extreme to another in relation to the breathing effect. Before they work out, they spend the day in a total slouch. Once they start their exercise, they go almost into a military-style position, remaining completely upright, which is just as restrictive in its own way.

'The secret is to be comfortably relaxed and at ease, so that all channels of energy are opened. This way you turn your system into a fitness machine and discover that the best gym in the world is under your skin.'

So how do people get fit?

'Well first of all they have to get fit by making the decision to do so. It should not be a daunting challenge but unfortunately, because of the way gyms have gone today, people are often a bit overwhelmed when they see all the equipment and activity going on in them.

'They think, it'll take me ages to get to that level and because they feel intimidated, they lose their motivation.

'So it's a matter of deciding to do some simple things that suit the stage you are at in your life. You should start by doing something you can cope with comfortably but that will get you using yourself to get fit.

'So take a decision and act on it straight away. This will immediately cause changes in the system that will have a beneficial effect on the body. A lot of people aren't aware just how immediate this effect can be. They think that obtaining a certain level of fitness is about running a half-marathon or even a full marathon but obviously this wouldn't suit everybody.

'Many of my clients are people who wouldn't be seen dead in a gym. The whole fitness culture is totally off-putting to them. But they are willing to take the trouble to learn and practise good posture and breathing which they know will help them get fit. They might enjoy walking with the dogs and just being solitary. Often this is the perfect outlet when you have been dealing with people all day long in your job and you don't want to spend the evening in traffic or in a crowded gym.

'So you begin your fitness regime by starting to use the breathing apparatus in the body properly and efficiently. You start becoming aware of all the activity taking place in your life on a daily basis and apply this good practice throughout.

'A lot of people think fitness is being dedicated to three-hour workouts eight days a week but becoming aware of how you use yourself and putting those wonderful resources into practice is really what counts. It is up to you then to decide how far you want to go with this.

'Fitness isn't so much about equipment as about how we use the resources we have over the course of the day. My book, *Dynamic Health* (now into a third print run having first been published in 1997 by Marino Books) is all based on posture and breathing. My belief is that if posture and breathing are working for us, we effectively turn everything we do into a beneficial exercise. Anything else we do as regards workouts and activities simply enhances the beneficial effect.

'So for instance, if you are slogging away on the treadmill at the gym and your breathing is shallow, you are losing 50% of the potential benefits. Reverse it so that your breathing is relaxed and efficient and you will enjoy 100% of the potential benefits.

"So what we have to focus on is accommodating these terrific resources that we have, to pump huge amounts of oxygen around the body that will make the muscles – including the heart muscle – work very well.'

Does this mean David isn't a fan of hard workouts himself?

'Oh no. I love to sweat and grunt too but that's because I enjoy it when I'm doing it. If you can find something you enjoy doing, not just because it's good for you, you will find that it's nice to do it because you enjoy it.

'I am originally from the fishing village of Kilmore Quay in Wexford, so there's nothing I like to do more than put on heavy gear and sweat over the borough, wading through cow shite. I find that incredibly liberating, spiritually, mentally and physically. So enjoying the exercise you do also adds a terrific force to the whole thing and perpetuates the benefits that come with fitness.'

Why are people so bad at harnessing these natural resources available to everyone?

'That is the real dilemma. My clients range from twenty-year-old hurlers to grandads and everything in between. Most of them believe that you must beat the living bejasus out of yourself in order to get fit, because this is the culture that has been here.

'But the reality is that you don't have to dedicate yourself to long, hard slogs to feel well. Just use the brains God gave you and make your exercise a pleasant activity.

'I suppose with the life we lead today, we're sitting most of the time and we're often overweight and out of condition. Our posture goes out of alignment more and more until we feel comfortable in it that way. If we try to sit straight or stand reasonably well, it feels unnatural. But the fact is that if your posture is out of alignment, that puts a huge strain on the skeletal and muscular system, with the most basic problem being that you can't breathe properly. Even accomplished athletes suffer with this. Some I have worked with tell me that nobody has ever spoken to them about posture before.

'So training the breathing system is the foundation of every programme I do. I've seen changes come about in attitude too, because posture is also psychological. If you slump all day long, you're sending a completely different message to your nervous system and to everybody else as well from what would be the case if you had your head up, shoulders level. So physiology, attitude are everything.'

Could you not get the same results from practising straight yoga?

'I wanted to make fitness more accessible to everybody. The people who were never into fitness, they're exactly the people I want to get hold of. It's not about being a fanatic. It's about simple techniques required to put breathing and posture into place and benefit the body overall as a result.

'So I get people to think, how am I breathing, how am I standing, how am I carrying myself, what is my voice tone, how do I sound to myself and other people? Awareness is everything. People I work with hate exercise but have learned about breathing and posture and put it into practice. One man of fifty-nine lost two-and-a-half stone. He went from being a workaholic with three companies to being fitter than he was in his thirties.

'It's not about long sessions at the gym. Somebody who has to run up stairs two or three times a day as part of his work, who does it with the right posture and breathing, using himself and all those natural channels to get the most out of this movement, turns this simplest of actions into a beneficial workout and makes a hell of a difference to how his body performs.

'Also, practising this system, people are a lot more relaxed and comfortable within themselves. Getting rid of tension in the body frees up circulation everywhere. The whole eliminative system works better, the digestive system, everything goes into active use. All we have to do is give the body the chance to do this and the alacrity with which it responds even to small changes is amazing.

'I often liken how it works to a pool at the bottom of the garden that has no inlet or outlet stirring up the water. So it just stagnates. After a couple of months, no way would you dip your hand in for a mouthful of water, no matter how thirsty you might be. But if you put in an outlet it will clean the pool out and there will be a constant flow in and out, just like our insides when they are fed with oxygen. So you're getting rid of muck and gunk. You can maintain this cleansing circulation on a continual basis once you practise getting your posture and breathing correct. So they are skills and it's all about practising them, and being aware.'

What about nutrition and diet?

'Yes, I'm a dietician as well and good nutrition is absolutely vital. The old cliché that you are what you eat is perfectly correct. Every cell in our body must have two essential things – oxygen and the right kind of materials to flourish. The great thing is we have a huge amount of control over both. We can make sure our lungs are processing adequate oxygen into the cells just by becoming aware of it. We can also make beneficial dietary changes if we're conscious about food. Diet doesn't have to mean deprivation. Just use the proper food and get it to work for you.'

How do people begin this dietary overhaul?

'Start by looking at your weekly shopping. The amount of stuff we put into our baskets and trolleys that are sugar, fat, additives and practically nothing else, is astonishing. The great irony is that most of us are overfed but undernourished in the western world. Research has shown us that people lying in hospital suffering from malnutrition are often overweight.'

What foods should we be eating?

'This is something people instinctively know but for some reason they choose not to do. The essence of a good diet is to use live or whole foods as much as possible, that is vegetables and plant-based foods that grow in the ground, alongside nourishing proteins and meats such as chicken and fish. So it is back to the basics that Mum and Dad reared us on. We should also drink reasonable amounts of water to stay hydrated but don't flood yourself with the stuff.

'We need to make serious inroads into our use of processed food and cut back severely on these. They are just habits. I've worked with people who've lived on tea and chocolates and who swear they couldn't have a cup of tea without the biscuits. But it's not natural to eat this way, even if it may be 'normal' because we're conditioned that way.

'Once people become aware of making changes, they find it isn't that hard after all – it was just habit. So it's about deciding to make changes in the first place. The one other essential I would recommend in the diet is a good multivitamin supplement, because most foods today are nutrient-deficient.'

Why do you say people should be fit in order to succeed?

'Whatever aspiration we have in life, whether it is to keep the house tidy or run a multi-million pound corporation, we just can't function well if our bodies aren't physically in good order. We are the instruments of our own activity, so it is we who decide whether to spend our time sitting behind a desk or a little bit of time on our feet keeping the body active.

'The reality is, whatever I aspire to, I will only be as good as the condition I'm in. Your attitude and how you feel emotionally about it will influence how you perform. If we're in good condition we can use all our natural resources to their greatest potential but if we're not in good condition, we can do damn all.'

You say we are our own greatest asset – what does this really mean?

'If we have things we want to achieve or contributions we want to make, we can realise them if we're in condition and have the drive and the will to do so. Most of us do actually have that drive but, unfortunately, do not realise we have it because we're not able to use it. So we let our natural drive dissipate through fear and tension and allow ourselves be distracted from what we really want to do in our lives.

'It is very important to be in good shape mentally, to know what we want and where we're going. We also need to be able to switch off the emotional energy that goes with activity when necessary and begin to pace ourselves. By doing so, I believe we can make the most of ourselves and harness our talents for a much more fulfilling life.

'If we're tired, run down and out of shape, even getting out of bed in the morning is difficult. But if we get out of bed with energy and enthusiasm, we set ourselves up to achieve.

'It's a terrible reflection on our society today that phrases such as "Thank God It's Friday" have become part of the norm. Very few say, "Thank God it's Monday," even though going to work with a sense of anticipation is exactly how people should feel at the start of each week.

'I do a fair bit of work with companies around the city and I often ask clients how they feel about their job, getting up at 7 o'clock on Monday to start off the week?

'Ideally, I would like to hear them reply that they regard this weekly early-morning start as a great opportunity to use a new week to achieve some things they want to achieve; that they see it as yet another chance to develop themselves and be of use to themselves and the business they are involved in. So what they really should be saying is that every Monday morning brings a great new opportunity for them.

'Of course, this is not what I hear. Instead, the reply is generally, "Oh God, another Monday morning to me means the weekend is over." Then they put their head in their hands and ask, "What on earth will we do until next weekend?"

'I work on a one-to-one basis with most clients so it's easier to harness motivation in people with this approach. Usually, I talk to people on the themes of how to have energy for life, happiness and success. This boils down to telling people that whatever they chose to do in life, they should commit to doing it well.

'For example, as I am talking right now, there is a man cleaning the street below me. He is making it really clean, so his work is a great success. Now if that same man had enjoyed the good fortune of a third-level education, he would probably be running a company and making a success of that as well, because his attitude towards his work is good.

'The mistake people have been making in the last ten to fifteen years as a result of the Celtic Tiger is that they think success is about material things. But success is actually about achieving what you set out to do. If we set out to make a success of a single day or to improve a service to a client and if we achieve that, we've succeeded for that day.

'Or if I decide I'm going to have a better relationship with my partner today and I go on to achieve that, that is a success. Sometimes we overlook these simple successes because we haven't made a million or we don't yet drive a Ferrari. But a success is a success.'

How do people find goals?

'Some people might say that they can't make goals because they don't have goals in life but this is simply not true. They need to realise that everybody has a goal, even if it's not one that is focused on the career ladder. For instance, a guy bombed out of his head on joints has achieved his goal of oblivion! So you're only fooling yourself if you think you don't have any goals.'

Why are people so stressed today?

'Stress is huge among people at all levels of society today. Even kids are under stress with the standards of education they are expected to achieve. We all have different levels of existence but I don't know whether we are adapting to the stresses in our lives that readily.

'Fundamentally, we need to be physically fit to cope. One of the ways we can manage the stress in our lives is by developing awareness of when we are getting into states of anxiety. Once we acknowledge that this is happening, it's astounding what we can do about it. Very simple relaxation techniques and developing some strategy to see the stress for what it is will help us to get through it.

'Not a lot of people recognise stress for what it is. It is something very insidious that creeps up on us, affecting our wellbeing in a negative way. But people are confused about this, as stress nowadays is often associated with the positive, reflecting effort and achievement. So we think that if we're not stressed, we mustn't be trying hard enough.

'If people consciously allow themselves to be more relaxed, they will find they have more natural resources available and can achieve better results.

'Champion athletes are the perfect example here. Some of these, who are on top of their game, are often noteworthy for how relaxed and completely focused they look when a good performance is crucial. This is because they don't have the distraction of stress to take away from scoring a goal or sinking a putt. They are not fussed or stressed about it because they know they are free to do it and have the ability to do it and that is exactly what they do.'

What does it mean to be fit?

'Being fit is about having your system working the way nature, and maybe your God intended. The lives we live today are very sedentary. We weren't designed to sit around slumped in front of the TV or computer. What we were designed for was to be active and well and that is the beauty of it. We are supposed to be active and well. So when we do things that involve moving the body, the body responds. There is a difference in how we function, how we react to things. We think more clearly and don't panic or get stressed.

'Once our body becomes accustomed to being fit, our productivity often goes through the ceiling. People may not see immediate tangible effects with regard to money over the counter in their business or growth in turnover but the managers in a lot of companies I work with know that having a fit staff improves the overall environment. People work better individually and respond more readily as a team to problems and challenges.

'Where people have learned to use themselves properly, particularly in the world of sales, they have been able to turn their lives around. While you may be well versed in selling techniques, if the instrument used to express them, that is, you, is run down, burned out or fatigued, you simply can't perform.

'Let's face it, when people think of getting fit, most people think it is something that requires hour-long workouts several times a week. Well, I work out three times a week for between twelve and fourteen minutes at a time. The exercise is incidental to my breathing and posture habits and my ongoing awareness of these, because maintaining good posture and breathing lets the system function in a way that is helpful to us. Breath-work in general and doing whatever exercise you do with some degree of enjoyment – that is what will keep you fit. So you don't have to spend hours and hours slogging away. That's what I've been preaching for the last forty years and that is what I will continue to preach, especially now when people need to be fitter than ever to get through the current global recession.'

Further information on David can be found at www. davehegartysdynamichealth.com or at Dynamic Health, 53 Middle Abbey Street, Dublin 1; telephone 01-8723080.

9

Expert Sporting and Fitness Tips

In this chapter three fitness experts share their thoughts on how exercise and keeping active can enhance the quality of our lives. Former Irish running champion, Catherina McKiernan, sports doctor Frank Brennan and personal trainer Paul O'Brien all speak convincingly about the health benefits of exercise.

CATHERINA'S CHI RUNNING
Some runners just like to run while others want to run better. Fortunately there is now an excellent running coach in Ireland in the person of former champion athlete Catherina McKiernan, who specialises in a technique called 'chi running'.

Catherina runs her own business, coaching runners in this technique, and from small beginnings, the programme is in huge demand.

Catherina, who was born in 1969, excelled at track and cross-country events since winning the Irish Schools' Cross-Country Championship back in 1988. She maintains that simplicity, routine and exercise remain her most basic tools for success.

Between 1992 and 1995, she won the silver medal in the World Cross Country Championships four years in a row and represented Ireland at the Olympics in 1992 and 1996.

She then moved into distance running, securing the best time for a first-time marathon runner in Berlin in 1997, when she set an Irish record of two hours twenty minutes and forty-four seconds. She went on to win the 1998 London Marathon – the first Irish person to do so. In the same year she ran the Amsterdam Marathon in two hours twenty-two minutes and twenty-three seconds, which remains an Irish record.

A native of Cornafean, County Cavan, Catherina remains true to her farming background, sticking to life-long routines that include an early-to-bed policy, clean living and plain food.

Since officially retiring as a competitive athlete in 2004, she has been specialising in coaching chi running, which promotes efficient and effective running by combining work on posture, core muscle usage and elements of Tai Chi. Her autobiography, *Running for My Life*, was published in 1995 and provides a riveting account of just how determined athletes must be in order to achieve their goals.

'I still run every day for about an hour, usually early in the morning, and I still love to get to bed at ten every night if I can. I go to sleep looking forward to my run the next day.'

The chi running programmes take place every weekend and Catherina recently introduced aqua running sessions but she says she doesn't let them take up 'too much of her time'. She also insists that she would never, ever, regard herself as a 'businesswoman'.

'No, I could never be a businesswoman. That is not how I

see myself now. All I am doing is teaching people something I love and have always loved. Knowing I am helping people gives me huge satisfaction.'

Catherina's courses are held at the Castleknock Hotel and Country House, which is convenient to the sprawling Phoenix Park – perfect for the chi running training sessions.

When I first approached Catherina with a view to gaining some insight into her running life and her more recent success as a chi running instructor, she readily agreed to help me with material for this book.

Catherina acknowledges that keeping active and fit provides her with the tools she needs to stay on top of her own life. Since becoming a mum of two and launching her chi running training programmes, she has managed to maintain her fitness. She admits that she doesn't know what it is to be unfit, never having been in such a condition, unless temporarily as a result of injury. She has been active all her life. Running and playing sports were simply a means to make use of her high energy levels. She wouldn't know what to do with herself if she wasn't active, she explains.

When Catherina invited me to attend one of her courses to see exactly what chi running was all about, I took her up on the offer in the hope that it would help with my own marathon training. I learned that Catherina's weekend courses (which are booked up two months in advance) are in constant demand by companies, groups and individuals who want select/one-to-one coaching or follow-up training in chi running.

In the flesh, it is interesting to note that Catherina appears even slighter and thinner than she does on TV. She is relatively tall and strong-looking but her limbs are thin and sinewy. She carries absolutely zero body-fat anywhere – even after two children – and her legs are thin, yet powerful looking.

Watching Catherina move gracefully about is like seeing art in motion. She has absorbed the elements of perfect posture and minimal body tension into her everyday walking movements, so that even her manner of standing looks skilful.

Over the course of the day, Catherina put the nine of us who were attending the course through our paces as we practised how to stand, walk and then run with perfect posture. It may seem hard to believe that learning to stand properly can be so time-consuming but the truth is that it takes a lot of practice to get it right.

According to Catherina, there is a whole range of things to consider in order to master the correct stance:

'Starting with the head, you should imagine the crown is being pulled upwards towards the sky by a string – then keep it held like that. The neck should be nicely stretched out as well, with no tension anywhere.

'The shoulders, hips and ankles should be perfectly aligned, with the shoulders directly over the hips and the hips over the ankles. If you rotate your head downwards, without jutting it forward, you should be able to see the laces on your shoes. (If you can't, either your stomach is too big or you're arching backwards too much.)

'In the abdomen, the muscle triangle that stretches between the hips and down to the sacrum should be the only tense part of the body. This muscle band should be contracted at all times, but not in a forced way.

'The line of the whole body should be nice and straight, with the chest leading the way. It may feel like you are leaning the body forward but just look at your reflection in the mirror and you will see that what may feel like a forward lean is actually correct, linear posture.

'The ankles should be kept nice and loose at the front, with the feet fully on the ground. Walking and running should take place in a nice, easy rotation of one foot after another. It is very important that you land each step in the middle of your foot and not on the heel.' (Apparently landing on the heel is one of the biggest problems in running and runners who heel-run are placing added pressure on themselves as each step jolts the body into stopping momentarily. Over time, heel-running also leads to injuries.)

'To counteract heel-running, runners should focus on pushing off from the toes with every stride. This adds extra zest to your flow as well as being much easier on the body.'

Finally, Catherina taught us to keep the chin tucked in and carry a little bit of contraction of the muscles from the lower abdominals down to the pelvis as we ran, keeping the knees soft, the glutes soft and feeling nice and tall with the body evenly distributed: 'Be aware of the lower dip in the small of the back and ensure it always feels nice and relaxed, with no tension.

'It's all just practice until you get the feel of it. You will learn eventually to isolate the lower abdominals and let everything else relax. It may feel awkward for a while but then it will start to feel more natural. This is because it can take a muscle up to forty days to remember a new way of moving.'

In summary, Catherina explained that chi running is all about making that activity more enjoyable and effortless by incorporating good mechanics which in turn prevent injuries.

In her classes she focuses on key areas.

'Posture is the most important part. Without good posture, your running will cause you fatigue, misalignment and eventually pain. I do simple drills and exercises to get people familiar with good posture: to lean forward as a unit from your ankles so that gravity pushes you forward, as opposed to leaning from your legs; then pushing off from your feet as opposed to your toes, with gravity propelling you forward all the time.

'Then I do another drill of a good arm swing. It's amazing how many don't know what to do with their arms when they're running. After that I do some drills of good running technique, using video analysis to show people how to change their running form.'

Catherina had many other excellent tips to offer and spending time in the company of a running expert of her calibre was a wonderful experience for someone like me who is passionate about the sport. The biggest bonus I took away from the course was discovering, through the video footage, that my arms tend to drop as I run. The correct method, according to Catherina, is to hold the arms at right angles and move them forward and back from the waist, with wrist and elbow alternating at the waist.

Practising this on my first run after the course, I found it quite tough to push my wrists right back to the waist as recommended. However, my running time was quicker than before and keeping my arms diligently at right angles resulted in my shoulders dropping too, which was terrific. My general tendency was to hike up my shoulders tensely just before setting off running but I don't have this problem any longer.

Catherina also recommends you pump your arms upwards from waist to chin when tackling a tough hill. This was a completely new but beneficial approach. It was great to remove the attention from the bottom half of the body and shift more of the work to the top part.

All in all, my running became a more balanced affair as a result of my chi running workshop

Running has always come naturally to Catherina McKiernan, which makes it difficult for her even to remember a time when she wasn't moving her body or racing around from place to place.

'I always ran because I loved it. Then I discovered I was good at it when I started winning competitions. I can never remember being unfit. From a very young age, even if I wasn't running, I was moving.

'I remember one Christmas morning when I was very young getting on my bike and cycling for two hours. That was just natural. I did my fair share of work on the farm but I was always thinking what exercise I would do next.

'We lived up a long lane and I would usually get off at the bottom, leave the bike and run around the football pitch for half an hour. I don't know why I was doing it. Nothing was ever thought of it. My poor mother just knew I was gone, sometimes for four hours at a stretch, off exercising in a remote part of Cavan.

'I suppose I had a lot of energy and I just loved doing it. I was fit and active and it was all for the love of doing it. I played a lot of camogie when I was young. Before training I would often puck a ball around for an hour or so and I would be there then until 10 pm, the last to leave.

'I remember too when we went back to school in September

and I had to cut back on running because the evenings were getting darker. My sister had a lamp for her bike and I would get her to cycle the dark country roads so that I could run alongside her. In school I still ran and played camogie.

'I would hate it if I couldn't run. I know I would feel very down. There were various stages in my running career when I couldn't run because of injuries and that was a very depressing time. The drug, the adrenaline, I didn't like life without it. But I would cross-train then, using the stationery bikes.

'With injuries, I cried for the first couple of days and then I had to come to terms with it. A couple of times I wasn't that upset because I knew I was physically and mentally fatigued.

'I have no fear of permanent injury now because I know the way I run is more efficient and economical. If I had known about chi running during my running career I would have saved myself a lot of disappointment, frustration and grief. I probably had a good style of running when I was younger but I think the years of training – I remember particularly after bounding exercises were introduced to my regime – changed my style a bit and put me up on my toes, which is not efficient for distance running. The fact that my style changed over the years caused me some problems.'

It was after Catherina left competitive running after her last race in October 2005 that chi running entered her life.

'Our son, Patrick, was born in October 2006. A year after that my friends were away in America and they got the book on chi running by its founder, Danny Dreyer. I eventually plucked up the courage to ring Dan and asked to train as an instructor. I went to the States the next spring for the first time, then travelled over for two weeks and two weeks again to continue the instructor course and take the exams. There were also some workshops here and in London.'

Although following this new direction, Catherina, who is married to RTÉ reporter Damien O'Reilly, with whom she has two children, Deirbhile, six and Patrick, two, still didn't have anything specific planned for when she retired.

'I knew I wanted to have another baby but other than that I never really thought too far ahead in my life on anything.'

Developing the chi running courses was a natural progression over time.

'This is a business that is easy for me, dealing with runners and people who want to run. It's great doing the courses. I meet a lot of lovely people and thankfully there is good feedback. I hardly advertise at all. I get people by word of mouth and from clubs.

'But I do enjoy running my business. There are lots of e-mails and I always like to e-mail back. So there is a lot of administration and a lot of phone calls. I'd always have queries from participants after the workshops and that's grand too. It takes a little bit of time but it's still very enjoyable.'

No matter how positive a frame of mind Catherina keeps while running her courses, the fact that they are in constant demand can prove trying.

'Yes It can be demanding with a lot of people looking for me to go places, especially on Saturdays and Sundays because they are working during the week. Some athletes might have found they couldn't mix their training with having a social life with their friends but this has never been a problem for me. I'm not into the pub scene and going to bed early is natural to me.'

Catherina has always been naturally gifted with a high zest for life.

'I suppose I always had high energy levels. I remember my mother used to say, "Will you ever sit down, you'll kill yourself!" I just needed exercise to burn off the energy. Now I get more tired minding the kids!

'I'm still very fit and some days I run fast enough all right. Other times I think of relaxing and just having good fun.

'I run because of the feeling of wellbeing that running always brought me. This morning, for instance, before I met the group, I ran for seventy minutes. Sunday morning runs are usually a little bit longer than during the week.'

Because she can never remember being unfit, Catherina finds it hard to understand how people can bear not to be fit!

'I don't know how people can function without being fit. I really could not function if I had to get up in the morning and sit in the car for half an hour and then go into the office and be stuck there till 5 pm.

'The first thing I do every morning is get up, put on my runners and go for a good run. I love it. It sets me up for the rest of the day. If I didn't get out by the middle of the day I'd say I would have the shakes. I run in the Phoenix Park and see the cars not moving and I feel so sorry for them. Maybe they think I'm the mad one! They have other ways of satisfying their needs.'

DR FRANK BRENNAN
Frank Brennan is a Dublin GP and sports doctor who developed the i-step running aid.

According to Dr Frank:

'There is no doubt that keeping fit definitely helps you perform better in other areas of your life. Exercise is one of the many treatments that you can use for depression, for example, and research shows that even at molecular level it helps, because when you secrete endorphins – which is endogenous morphine – you experience a natural little pep.

'On a physical level exercise certainly helps but it helps on a psychological and emotional level too. Runners, for example, are by and large balanced and happy people.

'There's no doubt that some people who exercise too much are exercise addicts. I know quite a few myself. This is taking exercise to an extreme. I know people, for instance, who, on the day they got married, had a gym installed in their honeymoon suite. Like any addiction, when it gets to that level it is counterproductive. It's a little bit like over-training: after too much exercise, your performance decreases with time. Not only does your performance wane but your whole life becomes dependent on a particular activity, just as, let's say, with heroin addiction. So there is a fine balance. A lot of exercise is good for you but too much preoccupation with it results in it not being good for you.

'If it works and you're able to achieve a harmony in your life that incorporates success, then good for you, as long as it is not detracting from your life or your family life.

'I would recommend exercise for anyone with a career or who is in business. In fact I would recommend it for everybody. Business people are no different from everyone else but there is no doubt that if you are in business, physical fitness can help.

'It does happen that many successful business people do have very strict exercise regimens. Even Juan Samaranch, the former president of the International Olympic Committee, who is now in his late eighties, still gets up at about 6 am to do stretching and yoga. There are countless other examples of people in business who have strict fitness regimes and I am often struck by this when reading about chief executives of various companies in the *Financial Times*.

'In order to help them work and deliver in the fast lane of business, people need a lot of fitness; not just physical but mental fitness. The same applies to motor-racing drivers. People may not understand why these drivers need to be physically fit for the job but it is an extremely absorbing preoccupation. The level of stress on the body as you sit in the cockpit of the car doing lap after lap of highly-concentrated driving requires incredible fitness.

'I would say if you want to maximise your performance in anything, you need a lot of fitness. Parenthood is no different. To get the best out of your children, parents need to be fit. I can testify to this as I have three kids whose ages are one, two and three. I am reasonably fit right now and I know I use every ounce of my fitness to keep up with my children. On that level it is productive.

'If you want to maximise your ability to enjoy life and get through it, a fair degree of fitness is vital. It is probably not coincidental that people at the top of their game often tend to be very fit.

'I often say to my patients: if you want to live a reasonably long and happy life I recommend the hundred-point scale (but I don't have a crystal ball so don't blame me if I don't always get this right). The closer you get to a hundred points, the longer you will live.'

Points are awarded as follows:

1. Do you smoke? Yes – 0 points. No – 40 points.
2. Do you exercise? Yes – 40 points. No – 0 points.
3. Do you have a healthy diet?
    Yes – 10 points. No – 0 points.
4. Do you drink alcohol to excess?
    Yes – 0 points. In moderation. 5 points.
5. Do you take illicit drugs?
    Yes – 0 points. No – 2 points.
6. Is your blood pressure high?
    Yes – 0 points. Normal – 1 point.
7. Is your cholesterol high?
    Yes – 0 points. Normal – 1 point.
8. Miscellaneous (for example, too much sun).
    Excess – 0 point. Normal – 1 point.
    Top score: one hundred points.

'My advice is: don't smoke; exercise regularly; have a healthy diet and don't drink too much. We should also avoid being overly-focused on blood pressure – there is far too much preoccupation with it.

'Forget about your cholesterol. OK, I'm not saying nobody should be on blood pressure or cholesterol tablets but the focus on getting your blood pressure right can probably improve your life chances by, say, 1%, whereas not smoking might improve it by 40%. There are too many smokers worrying about their blood pressure whereas if they simply stopped smoking, this would improve their longevity greatly.

'We tend to focus too much on the minutiae and forget the bigger picture. If you smoke and don't exercise, no amount of cholesterol tablets or blood pressure tablets will make up for that deficit. There is an erroneous notion that if your blood pressure is under control and your cholesterol is under five, that's great. Far too many don't understand that the really important things are not to smoke and to do enough exercise. This message is just not coming through.

'There is one other somewhat discouraging point that people need to be reminded about. It takes an awful lot of exercise to burn off just a little fat. We are all guilty of overestimating the calories we burn off and underestimating what we take in!'

I threw some extra questions at Frank in order to gain further insight into his view of sporting fitness:

What toll does exercise take on the body as we age?

'Good question! In short, the answer is: very little. Exercise in general has a beneficial effect on our health as we age. It is good for strengthening bones (so less osteoporosis) and it's also good for our mental health (less depression). Like most things in life, too much of anything can be bad for you. For instance, it is not uncommon for footballers to have premature arthritic problems as a consequence of excessive training. The key word to injury-prevention is moderation: so frequent, low-impact exercise is generally good while excessive, high-impact exercise may be detrimental. This is why many runners instinctively prefer to run on grass – it's kinder to the legs!'

Why do we have to work so hard to sell the benefits of exercise to people?

'It is human nature to choose the path of least resistance and there is one thing for sure: exercise isn't on that path. It is quite disingenuous to say to those people who don't do any exercise that exercise is fun, because they know only too well that it isn't. Let's face it, exercise is hard – indeed, it can be very hard. Believe it or not, I am in agony two minutes into any run. I continue only because I know how good I will feel when I finish and that this feeling will last a long time. But for many people, that price is too high and they look for easier options. Unfortunately, there aren't any easy options.'

Do you notice that people involved in sport and exercise have a certain drive?

'I think everyone has the capacity to motivate him- or herself. The thing is that this drive is more obvious in those who exercise.'

What typifies a keen sportsman or sportswoman?

'Steely determination and a fascination with their own body image.'

Do being unfit and not working out make for an easier life?

'No. Modern life entails many commitments, so trying to squeeze regular exercise into a busy week is not easy for most of us. For those that do make the effort, the rewards are substantial. Exercise has both immediate and long-term benefits. Short-term benefits include an immediate feeling of euphoria due to release of endorphins and, most importantly, sufficient energy to get through the remainder of the week. Long term benefits include improved longevity and reduced risk of cancer, heart disease, depression, arthritis and obesity.

'One of the commonest complaints a GP encounters is a patient complaining of feeling "tired all the time". There can be many reasons for this but one frequent cause is simple lack of fitness. However, trying to convince the same patient that doing more exercise will result in less fatigue is not so easy. It usually boils down to motivation and, in the end, people with motivation will break free from the shackles of exhaustion.'

Is strength/resistance/weight training suitable for everyone?

'As a rule, yes I would recommend weight training for

everyone. It strengthens bones and tones muscles – hence the saying: a strong back knows no pain. To understand the benefits of resistance training, it helps to understand what happens to our bodies without it. Astronauts who spend a few months in the gravity-free environment of space have legs like jelly upon their return to Earth, which is why you often see them being carried from the space capsule. So our bodies need continuous resistance (gravity) in order to maintain sufficient strength and avoid bone or muscle wasting. And the key to increasing strength is gradually to increase the resistance on our bodies.'

What exercises would you suggest people do at a minimum?

'It depends on the age-group of course: walking a little every day may be sufficient for the elderly while it would be recommended for younger people to do at least one hour's walk a day, six days a week.'

Do people control their own destiny by the lifestyle they choose?

'By and large, yes. Of course, there are many factors that shape our individual destiny: education, wealth and upbringing are just some of the more obvious examples. In addition, a healthy lifestyle is likely to enhance one's life (and the opposite is also true). I'm stating the obvious here but healthy people can do more than unhealthy people. I remember one occasion where a medical colleague and I went to hike up a small mountain. When we got to the top, he was in bad shape and very short of breath. He reached for his pocket and I assumed he was going to give himself a few puffs of an inhaler. Instead, he pulled out a packet of cigarettes and lit up!'

At what age should health-awareness training begin?

'I believe the appropriate phrase is 'from the cradle to the grave'. Children are always learning and this starts from day one. They may not say much for a few years but they're watching and learning and learning and watching. And in that capacity, they should never be underestimated. What you do and eat will have a major effect on what they do and eat so set a good example early on.'

How forgiving is the body of past wrongs or excesses?

'This is difficult to answer. It depends on how badly one treated one's body in the past and for how long. Having said that, it's never too late to change and while one is still alive, there's always room for improvement as long as one adopts a healthy lifestyle.

'I really do believe that smoking is the biggest harm we can do to ourselves. Drugs and excessive alcohol intake are close seconds. The list of disease associated with smoking is very long but the crucial ones are heart disease, cancer and emphysema. It's the last of these that I often emphasise to patients. Many smokers often have a romantic notion that they'll have a sudden heart attack and die a relatively painless death. Indeed this may be so but it is more likely that they will develop emphysema – a particularly unpleasant chronic lung condition. Imagine the feeling of always being short of breath – not nice. Just breathe through a straw for a few minutes and you will get an idea of what severe emphysema is like. And, as a wise man once said, emphysema begins with the very first cigarette.

'I am often dismayed by mums-to-be who smoke. I ask them how would they feel if, when the baby is born, I walked into the ward and put a cigarette in their baby's mouth? The universal reaction is one of disgust, to which I reply, 'Well, that's what you're doing every day of your pregnancy.' Some get the message but sadly, the majority don't.

'The dangers of alcohol are well documented so I won't dwell upon them here other than to mention the five Ls.'

The five Ls?

'Yes, how you can tell if you're an alcoholic? Well, if your drinking affects any of these five L's you have a serious drinking problem:

1. Liver – do you have 'fatty liver' or even worse, cirrhosis?
2. Law – have you ever been in trouble for (say) drink-driving?
3. Livelihood – does alcohol affect your ability to do your job
4. Lover – does alcohol affect your relationship with your partner or family?
5. Libido – does alcohol affect your ability to perform?

'The other major modern-day hazard is drug abuse. I'm not taking about injecting heroin – that's a no-brainer. No, I have serious concerns with 'recreational' drugs such as cannabis, Ecstasy, sleeping pills and over-the-counter opiate-based painkillers (for example Solpadeine). The dangers of these substances have been known for a long time. I have encountered many people with serious problems with one or other of these substances and all I can advise is to stay away from them all if at all possible.

'I am often challenged by cannabis smokers in particular, who don't see any harm in having the odd joint. I disagree.

Cannabis affects the brain in the same way that a mug of coffee affects a coffee table – it tarnishes it. The effect is barely noticeable at first but with time, the change becomes more noticeable. It may start as subtle changes in behaviour, mood or intelligence and end up as a serious psychotic reaction.

'One of my main jobs as a doctor is to educate, and practically everything I've said here is common sense. Unfortunately, common sense is not that common. I usually end such patient consultations with my *Titanic* analogy. I tell them, "I'm the radio officer, you're the captain and we're on the *Titanic*. There are icebergs ahead so you can either turn around or maintain present course and speed. It's your choice. You've seen the film – you know how it ends!"

Here are ten of Frank's maxims:

1. A strong back knows no pain.
2. It's okay to pig out, providing you work out.
3. There's no such thing as bad food, only bad diets.
4. Fad diets deplete mostly body starch and water – not fat.
5. It takes a lot of exercise to burn off a little fat.
6. Emphysema begins with your very first cigarette.
7. If exercise is to be effective, it really should be weight-bearing
8. Fitness is a combination of speed, endurance, strength, flexibility and skill.
9. If something tastes really nice it's probably fattening.
10. If you want to live a long and healthy life, start by not smoking, take regular exercise, have a healthy diet, don't drink too much and finally, never ever take drugs.

PAUL O'BRIEN

Paul O'Brien worked as a fitness instructor for a number of years before setting up his own business as a personal trainer and life coach.

An avid fan of sports and fitness all his life, Paul speaks authoritatively and inspiringly on the subject of fitness and success, attributing his own current peak fitness to a growth in demand for his services and his own productivity. In his youth Paul played lots of team sports before graduating to marathons, triathlons and weight training,

So, Paul, how important is it to be fit in terms of your health?

'I think the first thing to say about being fit is that it gives you more energy, improves your concentration levels and, most importantly, heightens your self-esteem and confidence. When you are physically fit you tend to have more belief that you can go out there and do things. You are far more agile mentally.

'If I relate it to my own life, I know the times I have been most productive are when I am fittest. When I was less fit, I was definitely less successful. I've always found that exercise gives me huge access to my inner power. When I did the life coaching a few years ago, that was like an extra spur because it helped to increase my self-awareness about what motivates me, especially in the field of fitness but also in my life in general. So I stopped doing the things that sabotaged my own performance, such as my tendency towards procrastination; saying "Yes" when I should be saying "No", giving away my time too cheaply and being a bit of a Jack of all trades instead of focusing on where my strengths lie, which is in communication, fitness and coaching.

'One of the most important aspects of fitness is the access it gives you to your own power. At the end of the day, having a commitment to your own physical fitness is pretty much like having a commitment to running your own business. You have to be focused; you have to get up every day and put the thirty-five to forty-five-minute workouts in; there has to be a structure to your day; and you must follow an overall game plan. The whole process of committing yourself to an exercise regime pretty much mirrors what you go through when you're setting up a business. They both require discipline so using one to complement the other is natural as the two go hand in hand.'

Paul thinks the notion of early-morning fitness starts, as promoted by successful people such as celebrity chef Gary Rhodes (See Chapter 1) is excellent.

'When you think about it, what a great way to start the day! You're left buzzed up afterwards, feeling powerful and ready for the challenges of the day. You know that feeling you get when you finish a good training session: you feel like taking on the world. By doing that daily, you're incorporating it into your psyche. That's such a great way to start off each morning.'

Paul is realistic enough to realise that no matter how fit you may be physically, there will always be tough times in business.

'I think fitness prepares you more for the knocks you're going to get, particularly if you are starting a business, because it isn't easy. I can relate to this from personal experience as I remember starting up my own business. Initially I thought it was just a question of, "Here I am, now give me some business," but it's much more than that.

'You have to do your market research and establish whether you have a market out there. You're putting a lot of money into it but initially there are no returns. You have to keep studying your market and create a business plan.

'Then there is the advertising side of it to deal with, getting your own business cards, and the networking, which is so vital. So much more goes into it than you would imagine, and you have to approach it in a very methodical and focused fashion. I got into the habit of taking one definite step every day, such as focusing on the marketing side and moving that forward. I also record my daily actions in a diary and that keeps me moving forward. I have the focus and energy to do all this because I am keeping up my fitness. If you have the mental and physical fortitude, you're much better able to deal with everything.'

Paul believes that had he not invested in his fitness training, he might not even be in business today.

'I know that if I hadn't been at peak fitness myself, I would have given up on my business. I would probably have gone to being employed by someone else because it is much easier to roll with the punches as an employee. You're taking on an awful lot going out on your own but I have learned that if you stick with it and keep yourself fit, your business will go from strength to strength.'

As a Portlaoise man who has made his home in County Mayo, what is it about this part of the country that appeals to such a fitness fanatic?

'I just love it here in Westport and have never been as much at home anywhere else. To me it is one of the best outdoor gyms in the world and I've trained outdoors all over the world, including South America, where I did mountain-climbing and Australia, where I did a lot of beach training, as well as off-road and hill running.

'Here in Westport I train a lot on the beaches and probably my favourite place of all to train is Old Head. It's got a lovely long beach for running and just lots of simple things that provide the perfect workout setting. For instance there are park benches where you can do various exercises and the little car tyre that kids use to swing off the tree is at the perfect height for pull-ups!

'Plus there are just so many other natural attractions in the surrounding areas, including Croagh Patrick, Mweelrea and all that wonderful country at the back of Killary. So you don't even have to join a gym.

'On top of that, I have two dogs, a collie, Jess, and another more recent arrival on the doorstep, a Jack Russell terrier. Jess loves running with me and is a great training partner. She comes up the Reek and is much faster than I am, which is great when I'm doing my sprints. She'll start behind me and then fly past. The terrier is more of a yapper. Sometimes I bring her, sometimes I don't!'

As a personal trainer Paul O'Brien not only talks the talk but looks the part, with a strong and fit body.

'I think that when you're in the business I'm in you have to look the part. There are personal trainers out there who don't look as fit as they should but at the end of day, the product you are selling is yourself. You are your own brand.

'When people meet me as a prospective personal trainer I want them to think: this guy looks the part. If I were a bit overweight I don't think I would be happy with myself or able to commit to the business. Even if I wasn't in this business, I would still keep myself fit because my approach to life is very much a holistic one.'

Paul has also been able to work on his spiritual side through his fitness. Exercising allows him to commune regularly with nature and appreciate the outdoors.

'I have a huge commitment to my physical fitness and to my spirituality. I struggled for years with who and what is God. My self-study and journey in life have brought me to realise that we're all God. God is within us all. We all have divine capability, which equates to being the best you can be and feeling you're living 100% of your potential. To me that is an expression of God.

'This is very much in tune with something we talk about in life coaching, which is life purpose. When you are living your life purpose, you are totally in line with your personal values. My top values would be health and fitness, spirituality, intimacy in my relationships, personal growth and self-knowledge.

'If you have a history of being fit there's no reason why you can't enjoy being physically active well into your seventies and eighties. I think a lot of limitations are mental. We don't really realise the power and the potential we have. That's not age-limited at all. You can be twenty or eighty and still have untapped potential. Fulfilment in life is all about tapping into that.'

Paul, who is thirty-seven, hopes to remain active and fit for the rest of his life.

'I hope to be active right up to the time I pop off. My ideal way to go would be out on a training run or out climbing a mountain, cycling a bike or clasping my heart. I don't want to go lying on a bed and wasting away. I'd much prefer to go doing something I love.'

Epilogue: Fitness through the Bad Times

While I was trying to finish this book a most serious event occurred in my life that made the task much harder: my husband Padraic was suddenly and quite unexpectedly admitted to hospital for triple by-pass surgery.

This event came as a bolt from the blue for both of us, even though Padraic had obviously been suffering with symptoms he hadn't spoken much about. While what happened next happened slowly in a way, it also seemed to pass in a whirl. Padraic was admitted to hospital and underwent a number of tests on his heart, which quickly established that his condition was critical. He was told he might already have suffered a heart attack and from a bed in a ward, was quickly transferred to Intensive Care.

Once installed there, he was strapped to machines and monitors that took readings of his heart and vital signs. We were told he would be taken to the Regional Hospital in Galway for an angiogram, which entails a dye being injected around the body to show up any blockages in arteries or other circulatory problems.

With Christmas coming in just a few days, this news threw our world into a spin. Padraic had initially gone to hospital for a check-up but now nobody could predict when he would come out again. It became a frightening situation of touch and go after the angiogram revealed three badly blocked coronary arteries requiring immediate surgery. Padraic was listed for a triple by-pass within two days and I honestly admit that when the day of the surgery came around, I fell apart.

All I could think of was the negative. I imagined my husband dying under the knife and in my mind saw our cosy little family set-up disintegrate. I would be on my own, with four children under ten to look after and they would have no Daddy while they were growing up. It was a nightmare and all I could feel was sheer terror. Everything froze in my body as I waited for the outcome and naturally, my world of fitness disappeared. Nothing mattered any longer. All I could think about was life and death.

During this horribly traumatic time, I travelled to Galway most days while family members living nearby generously took care of the children. Every day they were farmed out to various households and luckily they regarded this new way of living as great fun.

I made a point of not filling them in on the seriousness of the situation, telling them instead that Daddy had gone to hospital 'for a rest'. They were too young to understand the truth and I didn't believe in alarming them unnecessarily.

Fortunately, as I write, this horrible experience is all in the past. Padraic came through successful surgery in the care of an excellent team at University College Hospital Galway and is back home and able to work again. For a few days after the operation, though, things didn't look so good. Some complications made it difficult for Padraic to breathe properly again and it was difficult for the medical staff to stablise his heart rate.

In the end, a concoction of drugs and round-the-clock

care set things on the right track again although, naturally, Padraic's condition will need to be carefully monitored for ever more. We can't take anything for granted but we have been given a second chance as well as expert advice about how to optimise our situation.

My world of fitness dissolved during Padraic's health crisis. I went from fitting in runs five to six times a week to not running at all. It all simply stopped. There wasn't time to run. I couldn't even think about running. All I could think about was Padraic and whether he would get better.

For three weeks life stayed on hold like this. Christmas came and went. I got through Santa duties, prepared a family Christmas dinner of sorts (minus Padraic) and counted down the days until he was deemed sufficiently recovered to return home to convalesce. Of course, life didn't dramatically return to normal when that happened and, in a sense, by the time the new year of 2009 arrived, our lives had permanently changed.

But there was a gradual return to normality in regard to my fitness at least. As soon as Padraic came home, I started running again and the release I got from doing so was simply tremendous. Getting out in the open air, moving my body again, felt so good. After so many long days and nights of hospital bed-sitting, consumed with worrying thoughts, feeling uncertain about what lay ahead, it was a joyous relief to be able to think of nothing but getting air into my lungs. I ran and ran and ran. Day after day, as Padraic grew stronger and the feeling of life being on hold started to melt away, I realised that fitness training would get me by.

I have often reported on other people who claim that working out helped them through the tough times but I honestly thought they were simply referring to the natural endorphin high that comes from physical exertion. Now I was learning for myself that fitness training on an ongoing basis really does help you to cope with difficult life-challenges. Working out regularly helped me stay the course through Padraic's recuperation and gave me the space I needed to work out future plans – because, on a number of fronts, my future had never looked more uncertain.

Now that we have gathered ourselves again after our health scare, I continue to rely on my fitness training to help me to rebuild my strength and get back to work at my writing. That is the stage I am at now as I put the finishing touches to this book.

I hope you enjoy reading *Fit for Success* and that it provides you with inspiration for your own fitness and dreams of success.

I welcome any feedback to joangeraghty@gmail.com or editor@fitnessjunkie.ie.

Wishing you the best of health and happiness

Joan Geraghty